BELLY FAT BUSTERS for SENIORS

12 Weeks to Lose Weight, Gain Strength, and Improve Balance

PAIGE WAEHNER

Skyhorse Publishing

Skyhorse Publishing books may be purchased in bulk at special discounts for sales promotion, corporate gifts, fund-raising, or educational purposes. Special editions can also be created to specifications. For details, contact the Special Sales Department, Skyhorse Publishing, 307 West 36th Street, 11th Floor, New York, NY 10018 or info@ skyhorsepublishing.com.

Skyhorse® and Skyhorse Publishing® are registered trademarks of Skyhorse Publishing, Inc.®, a Delaware corporation.

Visit our website at www.skyhorsepublishing.com.

10 9 8 7 6 5 4 3 2 1

Library of Congress Cataloging-in-Publication Data is available on file.

Cover design by David Ter-Avanesyan
Cover photographs by Getty Images

ISBN: 978-1-5107-6966-3
Ebook ISBN: 978-1-5107-6967-0

Printed in China

Contents

Chapter 7. Warm-Up, Cooldown, Flexibility, and Core Workouts   77

Chapter 8. Weeks 1 & 2–Let's Get Started   95

Chapter 9. Weeks 3 & 4–Getting Stronger   103

Chapter 10. Weeks 5 & 6–Building Muscle   111

Chapter 11. Weeks 7 & 8–Making Changes   123

Chapter 12. Weeks 9 & 10–Getting There   135

Chapter 13. Weeks 11 & 12–Your Most Challenging Workouts   147

Chapter 14: What Happens Now?   161

Introduction: Getting Older and Gaining Weight—It's Not Inevitable

Remember when you were in your teens and twenties? If you're like me, you never gave a thought about getting older and how your body might change. We feel invincible when we're younger and never expect to feel anything different.

Fastforward 20 or more years, and a lot of things have changed in our bodies, our minds, and our lives. Just think how different things are when you get into your forties, fifties, sixties, and beyond.

Not only have your priorities changed, but you're no doubt dealing with many of the physical effects of getting older.

It's normal to slow down a little. After being alive for so long, we're bound to have the scars to prove that. You've probably had surgeries, injuries, chronic pain, and other damage that make your body hurt more or just get in the way of feeling good enough to exercise.

Another thing that happens as we get older is that our bodies start to change, particularly where we store fat. You may notice that you start getting more belly fat, and this can happen even if you don't actually gain weight on the scale.

Gaining fat around the middle happens to most of us—men and women alike—as we age. One of the main reasons for these issues is due to hormonal changes. If you're a woman in your forties, your estrogen starts to decline, sometimes it starts in in your mid-thirties. If you're a man, your testosterone starts to decline as well around the same age. These hormonal changes lead to a number of things:

- ✓ Weight gain
- ✓ Weak bones
- ✓ Depression
- ✓ Headaches
- ✓ Fatigue

- ✓ Brain fog
- ✓ Mood swings
- ✓ Hot flashes
- ✓ Difficulty sleeping
- ✓ Generally feeling like you spend most of your time entering a room and not remembering why you went in there

BELLY FAT AND WEIGHT GAIN

One study published in the journal *Climacteric* suggests that hormonal changes in women during perimenopause "substantially contribute to increased abdominal obesity which leads to additional physical and psychological morbidity."

Studies also show that, like women, men typically show increases in belly fat with age and decreasing hormones, putting us all in the same boat of more belly fat.

Women typically hold their body weight around the hips and thighs but, when you go through perimenopause and menopause, you quickly find that your fat stores shift right to your belly.

Men typically hold extra weight in their bellies, only adding to that extra fat as they get older and hormones change.

This can happen even if you've changed nothing about your eating habits or exercise routines, which makes it all the more frustrating.

Here are two things I want you to know if you're in this situation: You're not alone, and it's not your fault.

While scientists know we gain belly fat during menopause and, for men, andropause, it's only been in recent years that they've found out why. As the experts say, "Proteins, revved up by the estrogen drop, cause fat cells to store more fat."

What that means is that your body just naturally stores more fat without making a single change to your exercise and nutrition habits. Worse, you don't even get to enjoy that piece of cake or slice of pizza you passed up because you were trying to be healthy.

And how much weight you gain varies from person to person. One study published in the *International Journal of Obesity* suggested that some women can gain up to 12 pounds eight years after menopause. For men, one study found that, per decade, the average male gained about 3.3 pounds around the waist per decade. That adds up to about three quarters of a inch.

But, even if you don't gain weight, you may notice your waistline expanding as your hormones keep changing. Again, these are normal changes, but they aren't written in stone.

The nice thing is that there's something we can do about it. No, we'll never be our younger selves, that's just the way aging works. But we can be our best selves now no matter what's going on in our lives and bodies.

Learning more about what happens as we get older can help us make sense of what we can and can't control.

AN OVERVIEW OF HOW OUR BODIES AGE

We're going to get into the details of perimenopause, menopause, and, for men, what is called andropause to learn what happens to our bodies as we get older, but I want to pull back and focus on the big picture.

There are a variety of things that contribute to weight gain as we get older, things I'll cover later in this book in detail. But I think it's really important to understand that there are a lot of moving parts here and you can't always tackle all of them at the same time.

That's okay. We're here to figure out what's going on and how you can get started with a program that will help target multiple goals at the same time.

Here are just a few things that happen as we get older:

- ✓ **Hormonal Changes**—As mentioned before, estrogen levels tend to become more erratic, which may make your periods shorter, longer, or even skip months at a time. For men, waning testosterone affects sex drive, muscle loss, and more fat around the belly.
- ✓ **Stress**—As we get older, stress takes a strain on our bodies and minds. Chronic stress causes us to gain weight, especially in the belly, and studies show that aging causes oxidative stress way down in our mitochondria that can lead to damage in the body and aging.

✓ **Loss of Muscle**—We naturally lose muscle, something we call sarcopenia as we age, particularly if we don't lift weights. That loss of muscle is a main driver of weight gain because it lowers your metabolism so that you burn fewer calories overall.

✓ **We're Less Active**—We often have aches, pains, and other conditions that make it more challenging to move around more. One study published in the journal *Clinical Interventions in Aging* found that both men and women are naturally less active and have a reduction of functional fitness due to the aging process. This is due to loss of muscle strength and changes in body fat, flexibility, agility, and endurance. These are all things you can change with some commitment to exercise, and I've got your back on that.

✓ **Lack of Sleep**—Sleep disorders are more common as we get older. As we know, sleep deprivation not only makes us hungry for things like processed carbs, but it also triggers cortisol, the stress hormone that contributes to belly fat. Women and men may experience things like sleep apnea, which involves snoring and interruption of the breath, and women may have night sweats that interrupt sleep.

That seems like a lot to digest, but knowledge really is what you need most to make changes in your life. Patience, education, and of course the habit of exercise are all things we're going to work on.

I've been through this and I've had so many clients experiencing this very issue. It can be frustrating. It affects your self-esteem and your confidence. You want to feel good and look good, right?

This is so important to me because when I gained about 12 pounds, a lot of it around the belly, it affected every aspect of my life. As a personal trainer and fitness writer, I want to be an example to my clients and here I was, in that same boat as many of them.

It took some experimenting to figure out what worked and what didn't, but I learned a lot through experimenting with different types of workouts.

I'll tell you what the real secret is:

Resistance training.

RESISTANCE TRAINING IS THE ANSWER

Depending on when you grew up and your gender, you may have very different opinions about lifting weights. For women growing up in the sixties and seventies, it was all about cardio.

If any weights were used, they were usually tiny dumbbells that had us doing a lot of reps. Think Jane Fonda.

Men, on the other hand, were coached more into weight training and are, therefore, much more used to the idea of lifting weights than some women are.

Yes, cardio exercise is important, but adding muscle to your body is what makes the biggest difference.

If you're skeptical, let me share a few things that may motivate you to start (or continue) exercising and lifting weights:

- ✓ According to one study, 80 percent of people over 50 have too little muscle and too much fat. This is probably not a terribly shocking fact for most of us, but it's good to be reminded.
- ✓ There is a cause and effect relationship between losing muscle and gaining weight. That means the more muscle you lose, the more fat you gain.
- ✓ We may lose about five pounds of muscle every decade if we don't lift weights.
- ✓ Muscle is metabolically active 24 hours a day. If you lose five pounds of muscle, your metabolism drops about three percent. You burn fewer calories and those extra calories end up stored as fat.
- ✓ This metabolic slowdown can lead to an extra *15 pounds* each decade, which is crazy, I know.

To sum it up, if you're not exercising and lifting weights, you may lose *15 pounds of muscle and gain 45 pounds of fat over the decades.*

That's a lot and probably something most of us aren't aware of.

But, here's the good news: This is reversible at *any age.*

In just one study published in *Medicine & Science in Sports & Exercise,* experts found that, first, loss of muscle contributes to frailty and functional impairment. They also found that resistance training can help you gain muscle if you're an older adult. The bottom line is, you're never too old to make changes in your body!

Go with me on this journey. See how strong you can be. Feeling good in your body, being more independent, and feeling self-reliant will become more important than a number on a scale.

Chapter 1

The Basics of Perimenopause and Menopause—What Happens as We Get Older

To begin, we're going to delve into menopause because there are a lot of mysteries surrounding this process. I think we generally know what it is, but if you're like me, menopause was never discussed in our household. I think a lot of us are in that position, which makes it so hard to go through without knowing what's happening behind the scenes in your body. We're all different and some of us will have different experiences with symptoms.

I think it's important to shine a light on this so we can learn to embrace it rather than be afraid of it. While men also have a kind of andropause (which is when testosterone starts to decline), a woman's experience with menopause can include all kinds of symptoms, some of which we may not even know about.

One study showed that there are about 34 symptoms of menopause, although most of us won't experience all of them. Still, that describes how all-encompassing this can be and gives you a handle on what's going on with your body.

First, I'd like to share a quote that has helped me through this. It's from Lara Briden who wrote an amazing book, *Hormone Repair Manual: Every Woman's Guide to Healthy Hormones After 40*. She says:

"I view the body as a logical, responsive system that knows what to do when it's given the right support with nutrition and natural treatments."

That puts a positive spin on the process, right? And it's too easy to be negative as your body changes in ways you don't understand. That's where we're going here. We're going to understand what's happening and then we're going to figure out the best way to deal with it and, bonus, lose weight.

1

Let's start with the difference between perimenopause and menopause because perimenopause is a time you may experience lots of changes as well as more belly fat.

WHAT IS PERIMENOPAUSE?

Perimenopause is basically like a second, temporary puberty. Good times, right? It's a sequence of events in your body that starts anywhere from two to ten years before menopause, which is when you stop having periods. It can be a bit hard to pinpoint because it happens to women at different times and not everyone has the same symptoms.

As you stop ovulating, your hormones start to fluctuate, which can affect everything from your periods to your moods to, yes, brain fog. You forget why you go into a room, you may forget appointments, sometimes you may even forget to pay your bills.

This can start happening in your mid-thirties or when you reach your forties. The hard part is knowing when it starts and what's happening, since the symptoms fluctuate from day to day, even week to week.

It all comes down to two important hormones: Estrogen and progesterone, both of which are produced in the ovaries.

I know a lot of us don't really remember everything we learned in health class (if we learned anything), but here's a broad overview.

When you hit first puberty, progesterone goes up to prep your body for pregnancy. If you don't get pregnant, it goes down and estrogen goes up. This keeps happening throughout your life unless you get pregnant or end up having a hysterectomy, which puts you immediately into menopause.

During perimenopause, your hormones fluctuate, which is what can cause some symptoms you may be familiar with including hot flashes, night sweats, mood changes, brain fog, joint pain, and more.

And here's the thing about estrogen: It regulates a lot of things in your body. Building strong bones, controlling your cholesterol, balancing your moods, and preventing aging skin.

With that knowledge, it's no wonder our bodies and minds change so much in this time of life. You'll learn more about all of that later. For now, it's good to know that these are processes we all experience and they're normal.

You are not alone, and there are things you can do to make this time of life more comfortable.

WHAT IS MENOPAUSE?

Menopause is a little easier to define because it's basically when you stop having periods. Your ovaries no longer produce estrogen or progesterone and, while it's different for everyone, experts generally put you in the menopause category when you haven't menstruated for a year.

On average, this happens naturally by around fifty-one, but again this is just an average. Some women will go through menopause early, others later. It can be frustrating to not have a timeline, but you can learn more about how your body works and what you can do to keep yourself healthy and fit.

It really is a day-to-day process, and the act of accepting what your body is going through as a natural process can help you look at it in a more positive light.

WHAT AGE DOES IT HAPPEN?

That's a great question that no one can really answer and it's just one question I'm sure every woman would love to know. Unfortunately, there isn't a set time that it happens. Here's what experts in a study published in *The National Women's Studies Association* had to say:

> "Despite the growth of biomedical and feminist research on menopause, we still lack a comprehensive definition of what reproduction aging is, when it begins, how long it lasts, and how women experience different menopausal stages."

Well, that's a little disappointing, right? With that said, you've probably figured out that there's not really a great way to pinpoint where you are in the perimenopause/menopause journey. The average is about 45 through 55 years of age, though perimenopause can continue for years before you finally get through menopause.

I talk about many of the symptoms of perimenopause later in the book and how you can manage them, but it really does change from woman to woman. The important thing is that you *can* do something about any symptoms you're having and you *can* lose weight.

I'll show you how. Stick with me and let's go through this together.

HOW TO KNOW IF YOU'RE IN MENOPAUSE

If you suspect you're experiencing perimenopause, this is a great time to get an exam from your doctor. Keep a calendar of your periods so you can see if they're fluctuating. Your doctor can go over your history and signs and symptoms.

Unfortunately, there aren't any tests to make sure you're in menopause. Hormones change from day to day, so getting your hormones tested for that purpose isn't that reliable.

You have to get to know your body and, as we go through the symptoms of perimenopause, you'll learn exactly what's going on and some ideas of how you can deal with them.

Again, medical experts usually say that you're in menopause after 12 months without a period. Where I live, if you're having surgery, they automatically give you a pregnancy test even if you haven't had a period in two years.

And as author Stephanie S. Faubion writes in *The Menopause Solution*, "Menopause is not an illness. It is a natural part of life." That's a great way to turn your mind around and realize this is happening, we can manage it, and there are lots of options for what we can do about it.

It's hard to see the positive sometimes, but we'll get through this together and I'll show you exactly what to do to lose extra belly fat and stay strong.

THE TRUTH ABOUT LOSING WEIGHT DURING AND AFTER MENOPAUSE

There are a lot of things about perimenopause/menopause that contribute to weight gain as we get older, something we'll be talking about throughout this book. We've talked about hormonal changes and the fact that estrogen levels can lead to a variety of issues, one of which is weight gain.

Estrogen is just one hormone that helps regulate metabolism, one reason that we often gain weight as we get older.

Other factors we'll review include the issues mentioned before—lack of exercise, sleep disorders, stress, loss of muscle mass, and generally being less active.

The fact is that losing weight as we age is harder and it takes longer, but it's not impossible and it's worth it. What it really takes is this:

Taking care of yourself.

That means physically, mentally, emotionally, and psychologically. The truth is that losing belly fat requires some focus and some effort, but it doesn't have to take over your life. In fact, you'll find that the tips here are all about the small choices you make each day.

Granted, it's not as easy as it was to lose weight when you're, say, 25 years old. That's just nature and, frankly, a lot of us wouldn't be all that jazzed to be that young again. Maybe you felt good physically, without even realizing it, but life does get easier with knowledge and experience.

You can use the wisdom you have now to make a plan for getting yourself in the best shape you can. You've got the experience and the patience to make progress without stressing out about results.

A GLIMPSE AT WHAT WE'LL FOCUS ON

The things we're going to focus on include what I call the Big Five:

1. **Exercise**—Doing the right kind of exercise will help you make the most out of your exercise time. It's not the kind of exercise you may have done when you were younger. Science has advanced our knowledge of exercise, so we know a lot more about how to work out to reach our goals. For example, lifting weights was something a lot of women didn't do in the past. Now we know that lifting weights is for everyone and women don't have to worry about bulking up. We know how to workout to make progress, whether it's for losing weight, getting stronger, or being healthier.

2. **Nutrition**—What and when you eat at this time in your life matters, not just for weight loss but for your health. We'll talk about what you should focus on to lose weight and how to set yourself up for success. No huge changes, just small choices that make a big difference.

3. **Managing Stress**—Stress is a big contributor to weight gain, especially belly fat. We'll talk about how stress affects your body and what you can do about it. This is when putting your health first is the most important, giving yourself space to deal with all that life is throwing at you.

4. **Better Sleep Hygiene**—You can't always control the things that interrupt your sleep, but you'll learn better habits to wind down at night and give

yourself the best chance for a good night's sleep. This one is crucial and it takes some commitment to making better choices and giving yourself the best chance at good, quality sleep.

5. **Managing Your Insulin Resistance**—Your pancreas is in charge of making insulin, but if it can't make enough, glucose can't enter your cells which means that extra sugar ends up circulating in your body. That's a very simplified description, but it basically sets the body up for Type 2 diabetes. There are ways to manage this with diet and exercise and we'll talk about that and give you more information so you understand what happens in your body.

Taking time to take care of these things will lead you in the right direction. It may seem like a lot to take in, but it really is all about making better choices. You don't have to change every part of your life right now. That usually doesn't work anyway.

What we're focusing on are small things you can gradually introduce into your life to give you a leg up in the weight loss game.

In the meantime, let's learn more about perimenopause since a lot of us have never really been educated about what may happen and how to handle it.

THE SYMPTOMS OF PERIMENOPAUSE/MENOPAUSE AND HOW TO MANAGE THEM

For many of us, there's not much difference between perimenopause and menopause because they're all cut from the same cloth. Here, we'll talk about the variety of symptoms you may experience before menopause, so I'll cover the most common symptoms and the best information I can find on how to deal with these symptoms so you stay as comfortable as you can.

HOT FLASHES AND NIGHT SWEATS
Experts have estimated that about three-fourths of women have hot flashes, making it one of the most common symptoms of hormonal changes. For some, it might be short and sweet, while others might be putting their faces in the freezer to cool off.

Unfortunately, they can last for years. And then there are night sweats, which may wake you up in a pool of sweat. The weird thing is that experts don't understand the cause of hot flashes, but think it has to do with the part of the brain that regulates the hypothalamus.

There can also be some triggers that may cause hot flashes including:

- ✓ Spicy foods
- ✓ Caffeine or alcohol
- ✓ Smoking
- ✓ Being in a warm environment
- ✓ Stress
- ✓ And, of course, perimenopause

How to Deal with Hot Flashes

- ✓ **Figure out your triggers**—Pay attention to when you get hot flashes and make a mental note of any triggers like the ones mentioned above. Sometimes there may not be any specific trigger so you just have to ride it out. I do find that hot drinks and, sometimes, exercising in hot weather are definitely triggers for me.
- ✓ **Keep your core body temperature cool**—You may notice that your heat threshold changes as you get older. According to *The Hormone Repair Manual*, even the tiniest shift of body temperature can result in your brain making a temperature adjustment. That usually means hot flashes or even shivering. It helps to keep your environment cool if you can. Some women find that, after a hot flash or night sweats, they get cold as the sweat dries. It's great to have sweat-wicking clothes to sleep in so that you don't wake up in a puddle of sweat. Try www.soma.com for some great, affordable options for sleepwear.
- ✓ **Talk to your doctor**—There are hormonal treatments such as estrogen or progesterone therapies available. These aren't for everyone, but it's worth a talk with your doctor if you're having hot flashes or night sweats all the time. Keep your bedroom cool and use sweat-wicking sheets like PeachSkinSheets (https://www.peachskinsheets.com). There are also some antidepressants that can help with some symptoms of perimenopause, so that's worth a conversation with your doctor as well.

✓ **Exercise**—This won't surprise you, but exercise can help with many symptoms of perimenopause including sleep issues, depression, and memory problems. Studies are mixed on whether it helps with hot flashes, but some studies have found that regular exercisers had a lower hot flash frequency than women who were sedentary.

✓ **Breathe**—The Mayo Clinic also recommends practicing diaphragmatic breathing. Put your hand on your belly and take a breath. Your goal is to feel your stomach move out against your hand. Practice counting as you breathe in and out for four seconds. This can help you reduce stress and the chances of hot flashes. Try this in the morning before you get up and at night when you go to bed.

SLEEP DISRUPTIONS

Another common issue during perimenopause is sleep disorders. There are a lot of things going on in your body that may interrupt your sleep such as:

✓ Fluctuating hormones
✓ Night sweats
✓ Changing circadian rhythms
✓ Mood changes
✓ Sleep apnea
✓ Stress
✓ Nervousness
✓ Anxiety and depression

And that does not even include things like partners, spouses, kids, guests, and pets, all of which can interfere with your sleep.

Experts recommend we get at least seven hours of uninterrupted sleep. That's a great idea and one that I'm sure we'd all like to attain, but getting older doesn't always lend itself to more and better quality of sleep.

One study published in *Menopause* reported that up to half of women aged 40 to 59 reported poor sleep quality. That's a big number and one we can all probably relate to.

One of the big reasons we may have sleep disturbances is the fact that postmenopausal women are two to three times more likely to experience sleep apnea. Because their symptoms tend to be more subtle than they are in men, they may not even realize it.

Sleep apnea is a disorder in which your breathing repeatedly stops and starts throughout the night. It often includes

- ✓ Loud snoring
- ✓ Gasping for air as you're sleeping
- ✓ Daytime sleepiness
- ✓ Difficulty focusing
- ✓ Irritability

Usually it's a partner who notices many of these symptoms, which can be annoying. Take these symptoms seriously and see your doctor. There are a number of ways to treat sleep apnea including using a continuous positive airway pressure (CPAP), oral appliances, or other airway pressure devices.

My husband got a CPAP and it's completely changed how both of us sleep, so it's definitely worth looking into.

Getting Better Sleep

You've probably heard this advice before, but it helps to remind yourself what helps with better sleep hygiene. Creating the right environment invites better quality sleep and it all starts with a healthy routine including:

- ✓ **Exercise**—According to a *Sleep Medicine Reviews* study, experts found that consistent resistance training improves almost all aspects of sleep. It helps even more if you also do some cardio exercise along with your strength training. It not only helps with perimenopausal symptoms, it also helps with anxiety and depression. Because of that, strength training may be a very effective intervention when it comes to improving sleep quality. And, the great thing about exercise is it has so many other benefits as well, so even just a few minutes of exercise a day can make a difference.
- ✓ **Antidepressants**—There are a wide variety of antidepressants available and low doses have been shown to help with many of the symptoms

of perimenopause, including sleep issues. In one study published in *Menopause,* researchers found that some antidepressants significantly reduced the number of times participants woke up during the night. Be sure to talk to your doctor about this to find out if it's right for you. There are many facets to this treatment and you want to get all the information before you make this decision.

✓ **Hormone Replacement Therapy (HRT)**—This is also an option, which involves replacing the hormones your body isn't producing. The thing about estrogen is that it helps regulate your body's temperature, keeping it low during the night. When estrogen fluctuates, your temperature might be higher than normal, which can lead to hot flashes and night sweats. And here's something interesting as well: estrogen has a direct effect on your mood, acting almost like an antidepressant. It affects the serotonin in your body, which regulates moods and helps you sleep better. There are pros and cons to HRT therapy something you should research and talk to your doctor about as an option.

✓ **Better Sleep Hygiene**
   » Wind down at least an hour before you go to bed—as tough as it is, this means turning off your electronics. They often emit what it is called blue light, which affects circadian rhythms. This kind of light stimulates your brain, making you feel alert when you really want to feel sleepy. Make it a point to turn off the phone, TV, computer, tablets, and video games to get your body back into sleep mode.
   » Go to sleep and wake up at the same time every day. It's tempting to sleep in when you're tired and, if you really do feel drowsy, that's not always a bad thing. But your body craves routine, so try and keep the same hours every night if you can.
   » Avoid looking at your phone or TV if you wake up in the middle of the night—again, this blue light keeps you alert instead of relaxing you
   » A warm bath may also help you relax and unwind
   » If you can, try not to let your pets sleep with you. I've broken this rule many times, leading to cats on my head/neck/feet and me wide awake. It's great to train them when they're young to sleep in their own bed. I plan to take my own advice next time.

» Keep your environment cool.

» Reduce or quit alcohol.

» Try to avoid caffeine late in the day.

» Consider a low-histamine diet. This typically includes eating whole foods, fermented foods, foods that aren't processed, and other things I'll go over when we talk about nutrition.

» Consider taking magnesium, which can help calm your brain and reduce stress hormones, or melatonin, which helps regulate your circadian rhythms. Always talk to your doctor before you add any supplements to your routine,as they may interfere with other medications.

BRAIN FOG

If you feel like you can't remember things or you feel foggy, that isn't your imagination. Studies show that up to or more than 60 percent of perimenopausal women have reported difficulty concentrating and trouble remembering and retaining knowledge.

You know that annoying feeling when you walk into a room and totally forget why you came in there? That happens to a lot of us when we're multi-tasking, but adding the brain fog of hormonal changes makes it even worse.

For some women, this is mild and will eventually go away, but there are some things you can do to make it better.

✓ **Exercise**—As mentioned before, this is almost always the number one go-to to deal with perimenopause symptoms. It gets your endorphins going while sending more oxygen to your brain so you can focus better. Even a walk around the block can perk you up.

✓ **Get Enough Sleep**—Brain fog is always worse after a bad night. Researchers have found that sleep deprivation disturbs your brain cells' ability to communicate with each other, which can affect your short-term memory.

✓ **Eat a Healthy Diet**—There are plenty of healthy brain foods you can eat to help banish brain fog, or at least make it a little better. The big one is omega-3 fatty acids, which you can get from salmon or from supplements. You should also stick with healthy fats like avocados and olive oil as well as dark, leafy greens. You can easily mix some spinach or kale into a smoothie and you won't even taste it. I promise.

✓ **Exercise Your Brain**—Crossword puzzles, sudoku, jigsaw puzzles, and other games that engage your brain help to organize your mind. Not only is it a nice break, but it helps exercise your brain in a fun way. Even computer or tablet games can be great for your brain.

And here's something else to cheer you up. Dr. Gail A. Greendale from the University of California Los Angeles Medical Center says that you may feel foggy, but your brain is doing better than you think. "[W]omen still outperform men in cognitive brain studies at any stage of life."

It's not forever, so do the best you can by making small choices each day–take a walk every day, do some kind of puzzle for a few minutes in between other activities, and make sure you're loading up on brain-friendly foods. It all helps.

DRY SKIN

Here's another thing that estrogen regulates: the collagen and oils in your skin. That's why, as menopause gets closer and estrogen is declining, you may experience dry, itchy skin. Not only that, but your skin loses some ability to hold water, which also leads to dry skin.

This is something that doesn't really change after menopause, so it's a great time to focus on taking care of your skin and doing what you can to keep the dryness away as much as possible.

What you can do:

✓ **Wash with a mild cleanser instead of soap**—My favorite is SkinCeuticals Soothing Cleanser, but there are many great options out there at just about any drug store.

✓ **Moisturize throughout the day**—Experts recommend products that have hyaluronic acid or glycerin. That will keep your skin hydrated. My personal preference is CeraVe, which you can find at most drug stores at a decent price.

- ✓ **Wear sunscreen**—I'm sure you already know this, but you should wear sunscreen every day to protect your skin. Definitely talk to your dermatologist about what they recommend. I personally like Neutrogena products, which are light and work well under makeup.
- ✓ **Eat healthy fats**—I've talked about omega-3 fatty acids previously, those that are found in fatty fish like salmon. This kind of fat helps keep your skin hydrated. Other options include sardines, soy, safflower oil, and flax.
- ✓ **Eat more antioxidants**—This can make your skin stronger and, because these come from brightly colored fruits and veggies, you're also getting a healthy boost to your diet. Try blueberries, strawberries, dark chocolate (yes!), artichokes, and other berries to get the most bang for your buck.
- ✓ **See Your Doctor**—Your dermatologist is the best source of information for what's going on with your skin and will no doubt have great recommendations to get your skin hydrated and healthy. It usually comes down to the basics—staying hydrated, both inside and out, protecting your skin with sunscreen, and working on a diet that includes foods that are great for your skin.

WEIGHT GAIN

Of all the things that happen as we get older, one of the most troubling has to be weight gain. And part of that is the redistribution of fat in our bodies. It's true that fat migrates to the belly area as we get older, which brings us to the nitty-gritty of this program and what we're going to focus on.

It's important to know that weight management is harder as we get older. The metabolism slows down, we lose muscle, we're less active, and we continue to eat the same number of calories even though our bodies don't necessarily need them.

If you remember a few sections back, I mentioned that we could lose 15 pounds of muscle and gain 45 pounds of fat over a few decades. Thinking of those numbers is eye-opening and, even though it happens over a long period of time, it seems like it occurs overnight, doesn't it?

It's a creeping kind of weight gain, usually focused around the belly, because that's what hormonal changes do as we get older. Those changes redistribute fat to the areas we're least likely to have it.

Let's go back and remember the factors that contribute to weight gain and belly fat, including:

- ✓ Hormonal changes
- ✓ Loss of muscle
- ✓ Being less active
- ✓ Stress
- ✓ Lack of sleep
- ✓ Unhealthy diet

In several studies, experts have found that the change in hormones during perimenopause is associated with extra body fat as well as an increase in abdominal fat. I think many of us are familiar with this phenomenon. The question is, can we do anything about this?

The answer is, yes! And that's exactly what I'm going to show you in the rest of this book. Small changes in everything from your diet to your exercise program do make a difference. You just have to commit and realize you're important enough to make these changes.

Stay with me and we'll get there together. For now, you need to know more about what's going on with your body and mind during this period of time.

DEPRESSION AND ANXIETY

Unfortunately, another side effect of changing hormones may mean more symptoms of depression and anxiety. Experts say this occurs because of the imbalance between estrogen and progesterone.

When you get out of balance, you may experience mood swings along with anxiety and depression. All of this can contribute to sleep problems, brain fog, stress, emotional eating, and more things that also contribute to weight gain.

This is something you should see your doctor about. Previously, I mentioned antidepressants as a way to deal with some perimenopausal symptoms, but that also might alleviate your depression and anxiety. There are plenty of options available and lots of experts to help you navigate that process.

REDUCED SEX DRIVE

Another thing that may happen during perimenopause and menopause is one heck of a bummer: your sex drive may feel out of whack.

- ✓ As hormone levels decrease, it's more challenging to get aroused
- ✓ The hormone decrease can also lead to vaginal dryness
- ✓ There may be other things that affect you such as weight gain, hot flashes, night sweats, fatigue, and depression that can turn you off from sex.

So, what can you do about this? Again, your doctor is your best resource, but just some of the options include:

- ✓ **Hormone Replacement Therapy**—Again, talk to your doctor about this option if you're really suffering.
- ✓ **Exercise**—This will increase your endorphins and make you feel more confident in yourself and your body. We're going to focus on workouts designed to make you strong in every part of your body. That confidence will only help you feel more attractive.
- ✓ **Talk to Your Partner**—This can clearly cause issues if you're with someone, so communicating can help clarify how you can work on this together. A lot of us don't even know all the symptoms of menopause, and that for sure means that many men aren't aware of them either. Understanding what's going on physically and mentally may bring you closer together.
- ✓ **Therapy Can Help**—There are a lot of changes going on, and sometimes you need a neutral party to help you work through them. There are so many great therapy apps that don't require you to go into an office. Talkspace (www.talkspace.com) and BetterHelp (www.betterhelp.com) are two such examples.

The important thing to understand is that this can be a challenging time, but you can take control and do what you can to get the help you need. We all need support when we're going through changes, and having your partner's support is critical.

Remember that quote from before that this is not an illness, it's natural. You don't have to feel bad about it or dismiss your discomfort. It's hard, but we're learning more about it every day. We've got this!

WHEN TO SEE YOUR DOCTOR

Having gone through all of these symptoms and what to do about them, you may have a better idea of when to see your doctor. If your symptoms are interfering with your sleep, your mental health, and your daily life, that's the time you want to call your doctor and make an appointment.

I know we tend to put these things off, but there is help out there, so take advantage of it. There may be some small changes you can make that will make life easier. You have nothing to lose, and it really helps to talk to a professional.

And remember to see your doctor if you have any injuries, pain, or conditions that may interfere with your workouts. More on that later.

Chapter 2

The Reasons We Gain Belly Fat After 40

I've briefly mentioned the reasons we gain weight as we get older, and we're going to go a little deeper into that now so you can really understand what's going on with your body. First, we'll tackle the hormonal changes and go into detail about what happens to our bodies as we get older.

WHAT HAPPENS TO OUR BODIES IN OUR FORTIES, FIFTIES, AND SIXTIES (MEN AND WOMEN)

HORMONAL CHANGES

I've mentioned the hormones estrogen, progesterone, and testosterone, among others, and these hormones can start changing and fluctuating starting in your thirties.

For our purposes, we're going to focus on the later years because that's often where we experience the most changes in our bodies, minds, and lives.

Knowing what's happening is crucial for figuring out how to respond and realizing that it's not anything you're doing wrong. It's just a transition that we all have to deal with and we're all here to make that transition more transparent and easier to manage.

While we're all different, here's an overview of what happens as we get older:

BETWEEN 40 AND 45

At this age, women might start to notice changes in our cycles as well as other symptoms. Missed periods, hot flashes, night sweats, and the other symptoms listed previously.

This is the time when both estrogen and progesterone can start to fluctuate irregularly, bringing on these symptoms. Remember, these are the hormones produced by the ovaries and here are the major things they do:

- ✓ Keep your cholesterol in control
- ✓ Protectyour bone health
- ✓ Control your weight (yep, that's the big one!)
- ✓ Regulate your metabolism

There are many more functions involved, but these are the ones that tend to change the most in perimenopause.

BETWEEN 45 AND 50

This is when you might experience more symptoms along with the ones previously mentioned. This is because your hormones are fluctuating even more. You might have issues like mood swings, brain fog, hair loss, sleep problems, and more.

I do want to talk a little about thinning hair because it's one symptom I've talked to many women about. It's a little different than men in that we tend to have thinner hair rather than bald spots. This, of course, is because of fluctuating estrogen and progesterone.

One way to combat this is with all the things I've already mentioned: exercising, eating healthy foods, staying hydrated, and, as always, talking to your doctor about your options.

Not everyone will experience all of these symptoms but, if you do, it's totally normal. In Chapter 1, I talked about these symptoms and ways to handle them. You might want to look back and refresh your memory. Try to implement just one change to your routine. Let that become a habit and then add another when you're ready.

There's a lot going on at this time in your life, and it's okay to shift your focus to one area of your life and work on that. Trying to change everything at once usually leads to stress and, eventually, quitting.

BETWEEN 50 AND 60

Usually, by the age of 55 most women have gone through menopause. Remember those fluctuating hormones? They no longer fluctuate because, eventually, your ovaries stop producing estrogen.

Unfortunately, that doesn't mean you won't still experience things like hot flashes and night sweats. These can go on for months or years after menopause. I have a family member who still gets hot flashes even though she's in her sixties and has been in in the thick of menopause for years.

The key when you reach this stage of life is to focus on your health. Without estrogen, you are now at a higher risk of osteoporosis (bone loss) and heart disease. The good news is, you've got a way to defend yourself against these issues and it all starts with exercise. Yep. You knew that was coming.

The workouts I've created are just one line of defense against these things. Lifting weights will keep your bones strong and help protect your heart. And of course, as I will say ad nauseam throughout this book, you should always see your doctor. Have everything checked—your bones, your heart, your body, bloodwork.

The only way to be in control of your health and weight loss is to know exactly what's going on. It's tempting to avoid it, but that won't stop changes from happening. It's better to know what's going on and do something about it than to find out it's too late. You have more control over your health than you think!

BODY CHANGES IN MEN

Men also experience hormonal changes. These are different from what women experience, but similar in that one of the hormones regulating the body, testosterone for men, starts declining. This can lead to the following:

- ✓ **Gaining Belly Fat**—This can start around the age of thirty and can continue until roughly 55 years of age. A man's excess weight is usually carried as belly fat, which increases the risk of heart disease and other conditions. The good news is, if you lose weight, it usually comes off your belly first.
- ✓ **Loss of Muscle**—Like women, men's hormones decline around middle age, so you naturally lose muscle mass. The next section explains all about muscle loss, why it happens, and what we can do about it.
- ✓ **Heart Issues**—As men get older, the risk factors for heart disease and high blood pressure start to go up. Studies show that age itself is a risk factor for heart disease, but that risk can be compounded by things like obesity, diabetes, and frailty. These are all things we can combat with a

healthy diet and exercise . . . and, of course, you should see your doctor before you do anything to see if medication is necessary.

✓ **Prostate Issues**—The prostate tends to get bigger as you get older, which can mess with your bladder and make you urinate more often.

The good news is, there are things you can do about many of these issues by being healthy, losing weight, exercising, and lifting weights. We're going to cover all of them, but let's get through the rest of some of the things that can happen as we get older.

MUSCLE LOSS

I've mentioned this before and I will likely harp on it throughout the book because this is one of the most important factors in being healthy, independent, and losing weight.

Unlike some other issues that happen as we get older, we can actually do something about this one, so listen up!

Muscle loss, whether in men, as discussed above, or women, is also known by the fancier term sarcopenia. Sarcopenia is generally defined by loss of muscle mass as well as loss of muscle function and strength. It's also associated with gaining fat, which is one reason we might gain weight during this time.

In one opinion published in the *Current Opinion of Rheumatology*, experts suggest that sarcopenia is "one of the most important causes of functional decline and loss of independence in older adults."

Contributing factors to muscle loss can include:

✓ **Neurological decline**—This can include things like memory loss and mild cognitive impairment like the brain fog I talked about previously. We are also more at risk for strokes, Parkinson's disease, and Alzheimer's.

✓ **Hormonal changes**—Obviously this is something we'll be talking about all through the book, but estrogen and testosterone are muscle-building hormones so if we stop producing it, that can contribute to muscle loss and muscle strength.

✓ **Inflammation**—A study published in the *Journal of Neuroinflammation* (a little light reading for you) suggests that the transition into menopause (and for men with declining testosterone) prompts an inflammatory response. Here's the thing: Chronic inflammation makes everything worse. It causes stress and fatigue and is related to mood swings and sleep problems. It also contributes to insulin resistance. This can lead to weight gain. It's almost like your immune system is on all the time.

✓ **Belly Fat**—We've talked about how we gain belly fat as we go through perimenopause and to recap, it has to do with the loss of estrogen, lack of activity, poor sleep, and not eating the greatest diet. Wendy M. Kohrt, a professor of medicine at the University of Colorado, suggests that a complete loss of estrogen causes abdominal fat to increase by 10 percent in just five months. For men, they tend to carry their fat in their bellies so, losing that muscle and not eating healthy only adds to the problem.

✓ **Slowing Metabolism**—I've mentioned this, but our metabolisms naturally start to slow down, often in our thirties. The decline of estrogen in women and testosterone in men contributes to a slower metabolism. That means we're burning fewer calories which, of course, contributes to weight gain. The key here is that, because we can't really measure metabolism, we keep eating the same amount of calories, if not more, not realizing we're on the road to weight gain.

INSULIN RESISTANCE—FEELING HUNGRY WHEN YOU'RE NOT

For a lot of us, insulin resistance is not something we're entirely familiar with unless you have some form of diabetes. So what does that actually mean?

When you eat, your body breaks your food down into sugar, which starts circulating in the blood. Your pancreas then produces insulin, a hormone that helps move this sugar into your cells for energy or storage.

When your cells absorb that sugar, the levels in your bloodstream fall. When you're insulin resistant, your pancreas has to work much harder to produce insulin because your cells can't absorb that sugar so it continues to circulate in your blood.

This isn't something you know you have; you have to have your blood tested. But some signs you may be insulin resistant include:

✓ High blood pressure
✓ If your waistline is over 40 inches for men or 35 inches for women

- ✓ Skin tags which are small, soft skin growths
- ✓ High cholesterol

Being insulin resistant is associated with weight gain, especially belly fat. Exercise and your diet are your first go-to areas to help combat insulin resistance and belly fat. The workouts in this book address this very condition. Make sure you get a full workup from your doctor to find out how your body is working and whether you might be insulin resistant. This may affect your approach to your diet and exercise.

HUNGER HORMONES ARE OUT OF WHACK

We have a couple of hormones that help control how we eat. One is leptin, which is a hormone made by fat cells to decrease appetite. Ghrelin is a hormone that increases appetite and plays a huge role in body weight.

When we hit that certain age, the hunger-stimulating hormone, ghrelin, increases. That's the reason many of us find we're hungrier at this time in our lives, maybe without realizing it. At the same time, leptin, which is the hormone that promotes satiety, is reduced, leading to the urge to overeat for many of us.

As one article in *Psychology Today* puts it, "Menopause can make you hungry."

For men, low testosterone means less muscle which equals more fat, which makes it much more likely to be overweight.

When I first started researching this years ago, many experts blamed bad eating habits for weight gain as we age, for both men and women. And, of course, your diet is incredibly important, which I'll get into in the next section,

But, many women experience a change in appetite when estrogen drops. One study found that plummeting estrogen may account for 12 percent of women who are overweight in midlife.

Another study, presented at the annual meeting of the Society for Neuroscience, studied monkeys, which are very closely related to humans. They found that some monkeys increased their food intake by 67 percent at midlife. Obviously, that caused some significant weight gain.

This does shed some light on what's happening below the surface. These are things we can't measure—hunger hormones, changes in hormones due to age, lower metabolism, loss of muscle. It's not like we can know what's going on under the skin without help from a doctor or a lab.

We're all going to get older, that's a fact. And we can't always control the complex series of hormones fluctuating through our bodies. But, we can still control a lot, including:

- ✓ What we eat
- ✓ How much we exercise
- ✓ How we manage stress
- ✓ How we sleep
- ✓ How active we are

This is why resistance training is so important. Muscle is more metabolically active than fat, so the more you have, the more calories you burn. That's our goal here. We've also gone through all the benefits of resistance training which touch on the other elements contributing to weight gain and belly fat.

Resistance training helps you sleep better, reduces stress, and keeps you active. Your workouts are coming soon, and you can also skip forward to see what's in store for you or so you can get a leg up.

For now, we're going to talk about the most important and challenging element required to lose weight: your diet. As the saying goes, you can't out-exercise a bad diet and, believe me, I've tried.

It's much easier to cancel out your workout with something as small as a donut or a can of Coke. It's easier to eat more calories, since it's really hard to know what you're eating, than to burn more calories, since you generally burn less than you think and, again, it's hard to know exactly how many calories you're burning.

Thus, we're going to make it our goal to make some changes in our diets so we have the best chance at losing weight and being healthier.

UNHEALTHY EATING HABITS

After all of this, we now know there are many connections here between weight gain and hunger hormones that are out of balance.

We know that hormonal changes can cause all kinds of issues, particularly for women in perimenopause or menopause. In fact, *Medical News Today* suggests there are about 34 symptoms we may experience. That is eye-opening, right? Thirty-four.

We won't experience all of them, but just the thought of that many changes that could be happening can be daunting.

It kind of puts things in perspective as you try to take care of yourself. There are so many moving parts here, and there's no way for you to know everything. The best you can do is follow the science and that's what we're doing here. We're going to use what we know to get your diet in a healthier place and get your body strong and fit.

We're going to start with our eating habits, going in depth in the next chapter, but what I want to highlight now is the fact that hormonal changes do affect hunger.

There are other hormones that change as we get older, including a drop in serotonin, which regulates mood, sleep cycle, appetite, and even digestion.

With a drop in estrogen as well as serotonin, this combination, along with extra stress and fatigue we may feel, can cause cravings for carbs. Not all carbs are bad, but the ones we crave don't usually involve broccoli or carrots, right?

It's usually refined sugars, which are not great for our bodies.

When you feel tired all the time, your body is searching for energy, and refined carbs give you immediate energy. That's where those cravings come from.

Things like bread, pasta, rice, chips, and sugary treats may give instant gratification, but there's always a crash and then there's that icky side effect of weight gain.

We'll talk about your diet in the next chapter but, for now, consider adding more fiber to your diet and choosing whole grain bread, pasta, and rice.

Just noticing your cravings and writing them down can help you figure out your triggers and start to make some new habits. Probably the number one rule we use in our house is out of sight out of mind. If it's not there, I'm definitely too lazy to go out and buy it.

MORE STRESS

On another related note, all of the above combine to add to stress. We already have life stress. And then you add the physical and mental symptoms of menopause and andropause and you have the perfect storm.

There are more worries about getting older, frustration with weight gain, losing family members, and trying to figure out how to cope.

And here's the thing: stress contributes to belly fat, also known as "stress belly," although as you now know, there are many other factors involved.

When you're chronically stressed, here's what happens:

- ✓ Your flight or fight response kicks in.
- ✓ Your body starts producing cortisol, which is like an alarm system. Maybe there's no physical threat, but your body doesn't know the difference between mental stress and, say, the physical stress of our ancestors who had to deal with hunting and gathering while avoiding predators.
- ✓ We often stress-eat to cope when our bodies produce too much cortisol, but it actually redistributes fat to your belly to protect your organs.
- ✓ The result is often weight gain and, yes, belly fat.

It's so crucial to practice using stress management tools during this time. It takes some effort to change your habits, but you can do it. Think of it like brushing your teeth . . . something essential that you need to do every day. Some simple ways to start:

- ✓ **Move**—Set an alarm every hour and get up, stretch, move around,, or, if you can, take a walk. All of that gets your blood moving and gets you out of your head.
- ✓ **Breathe**—Even just one minute of breathing can reduce stress, believe it or not.
- ✓ **Exercise**—This is a great way to get out your frustrations and calm yourself.
- ✓ **Meditate**—Sometimes it's hard to do this when you're stressed, but practicing makes you better at it My favorite app for guided meditation is Calm (www.calm.com). There are so many choices for how to meditate, you can find one that fits your time limits and preferences.
- ✓ **Be Mindful When You're Eating**—Studies have shown that eating with awareness can reduce food cravings, better portion control, lower body mass index, and better weight management. Here's how you start:
  - » Eat more slowly
  - » Chew each bite completely
  - » Try at least one meal a day without any distractions like TV, smartphones, or computers. This is a habit you can build on over time
  - » Focus on the food you're eating. Maybe you need to make some changes to make healthy foods more enjoyable such as healthy sauces, marinades, spices, and dressings.

As a fast eater, I know this can be hard, but it's well worth the effort. Start small. Set a goal for one minute of movement every hour, one minute of breathing every hour, one minute of meditation a few times a day, and one meal where you're completely focused on eating.

CHANGING SLEEP PATTERNS

As I mentioned before, the symptoms of perimenopause and menopause can often interfere with sleep.

In one study published in *Menopause*, researchers found that "sleep efficiency was negatively associated with age, perimenopause, postmenopause status . . . hot flashes, and depressed mood."

What they looked at most was how much time people were awake in bed. And it's kind of a vicious cycle. You can't sleep because you're having hot flashes and that makes you feel depressed and/or anxious.

Then you have a lack of sleep, which can cause many of the same symptoms like:

- ✓ Memory problems
- ✓ Trouble concentrating
- ✓ Mood swings
- ✓ High blood pressure
- ✓ Weight gain
- ✓ Risk of diabetes and heart disease
- ✓ Low sex drive

Many of these symptoms coincide with the symptoms of perimenopause and menopause, so they are constantly overlapping and triggering each other.

Part of the problem is also a lack of *quality* sleep. Have you ever had that feeling that you didn't sleep all night, but you know you did? I think we've all experienced that sensation.

In the previous chapter, I talked about having better sleep hygiene. Things like winding down before bed, putting down your electronics, and keeping a sleep schedule.

You can flip back to that chapter for more ideas on how to get better quality sleep.

For now, I want you to understand why sleep deprivation often contributes to belly fat.

Remember before when I talked about chronic stress that increases the stress hormone, cortisol? Well, lack of sleep can trigger cortisol as well. Remember that cortisol increases the amount of belly fat, which is bad for your waistline and your health.

Lack of sleep has some other effects such as:

✓ **Lower Human Growth Hormone (HGH)**—HGH is a hormone that is responsible for growth, cell repair, metabolism, and body composition. Losing sleep can affect this, but exercise, diet, and losing weight are all things that can boost your HGH.
✓ **Compromised Immune System**—When you sleep, your immune system produces antibodies that help keep you safe from bacteria and viruses. If you don't get enough sleep, your body can't protect you as much.
✓ **Changes Your Hormones**—The hunger hormones, leptin and ghrelin, also change when you don't get enough sleep. This can lead to late-night snacking and insulin resistance.

Working on your sleep routine and doing what you can to create a quiet, calm environment in your bedroom and your head can make a big difference in weight loss.

NOT EXERCISING AND BECOMING LESS ACTIVE OVERALL

There is one more side effect of hormonal changes. When you think of all the symptoms of menopause like lack of sleep, hot flashes, night sweats, fatigue, and aches and pains, it's not surprising that many women are less active when they hit menopause.

On top of that, the metabolism naturally slows down as we age, contributing to even more weight gain. This is why exercise is so crucial during this time.

It helps your heart health, cholesterol, blood pressure, weight loss, bone mass, and reduces stress. It helps prevent injuries and falls that often come with getting older and losing strength, balance, and flexibility.

There isn't any treatment that improves all of these things other than exercise.

While the structured workouts in this book focus on improving all of those things, here's another aspect of movement that can add to your overall health and calorie-burn.

It's called NEAT—Non-Exercise Activity Thermogenesis. That's a fancy term for what I've been saying throughout the book, which is to move more. Workouts are obviously important, but many people have no idea just how vital regular movement is.

NEAT movement is a part of your total daily energy expenditure (TDEE), something we'll talk about more in future chapters. What's important to know is that any kind of movement, even if it isn't structured exercise, contributes to all the calories you burn each day.

One small thing you can do to increase your metabolism is to set a timer to remind you to stand up every hour, especially if you're working at a computer or sitting a lot. Just standing, stretching, and taking a short walk can get your body moving and contribute even more to your TDEE.

The workouts in this book will help you focus on all of these things. Most of all, exercise will help you feel good about yourself.

THE BENEFITS OF LOSING BELLY FAT

Of course we'd all love to lose belly fat, but it's not just great for how we look. It's also critical for our health. Let's motivate you even more by talking about even more positive things that happen when you lose belly fat.

- ✓ You feel and look better
- ✓ It reduces your risk of heart disease, some types of cancer, and diabetes
- ✓ It promotes better circulation
- ✓ It improves your sleep quality
- ✓ You'll have more control over your sugar

It's a slow process, but you'll feel the benefits even before you lose any weight. Remember the saying that it's the journey, not the destination? That's the mindset to latch onto now to keep yourself going. We're going to focus on the steps to take and how we can stay in the present and enjoy the adventure.

Chapter 3
Let's Talk about Your Diet

THINGS THAT AFFECT YOUR METABOLISM

As you no doubt know, working out is important. But . . . what and how you eat is crucial for being healthy and losing belly fat. This is where the real work can come in, but we're going to take it slow so that you have some tools available that make it easier to eat healthier.

Have you ever tried a low-calorie diet? I know I have and here's the problem: not only are you hungry, if you lose any weight it's most likely muscle. Remember that muscle is more metabolically active than fat so losing muscle means your metabolism is going to drop.

Metabolism is a very complex biochemical process that your body uses to convert food and drinks into energy. It all happens way down deep in your cells and many factors can affect it.

- ✓ **Genetics**—You've probably known somebody who could eat and eat and never seem to gain weight (try not to think naughty thoughts about them). Well, experts have found that those differences from person to person are partially due to your genes.
- ✓ **Size**—Studies have shown that the bigger you are, the lower your metabolism generally is.
- ✓ **Age**—As you already know, metabolism slows down as we age, but it's not something you can easily measure. We usually keep eating the same number of calories even though we don't need as many, which is one reason we gain weight. Part of this is natural aging, but it's also about eating less and exercising more so you don't lose muscle.

- ✓ **Body Composition**—To keep it simple, this is all about the ratio of muscle and fat. Muscle is the largest tissue in your body and it's more metabolically active than fat. Muscle can burn about 10 to 15 calories per day while at rest and contributes 20 percent to your total daily exercise expenditure (TDEE). This adds up to about four to seven calories per pound of muscle. Fat only contributes about five percent to your TDEE.
- ✓ **Sex**—If you're a woman, you probably know that men typically have higher metabolisms because they're often larger and naturally have more muscle because they have more testosterone. Women have more body fat and it all comes down to our hormones.
- ✓ **Health Issues**—Your thyroid is in control of your metabolism, so if it's low, your metabolism slows down and adds to weight gain. Diabetes can also change your metabolism. When your body doesn't produce enough insulin, you might gain weight, leading to metabolic syndrome, which includes having more fat around your waist.
- ✓ **Stress**—I've mentioned that stress can cause belly fat because of the stress hormone cortisol, which sends any extra calories you have right to your belly. You can revisit the previous chapter for ideas on how to manage stress. Exercise is always a good choice, by the way.
- ✓ **Dieting**—I'll dig deep into this in the next section, but one of the main culprits of belly fat is too much sugar and not enough protein. You'll learn what you need to do to start on the road to belly fat weight loss.
- ✓ **Activity Levels**—Very active people tend to have higher metabolisms than those who don't. Don't worry, though . You're not on your own. I'm here to help!

Put all that together and you have a metabolism that isn't working at its best. But, we can control many of these factors and that's exactly what we're going to do.

YOUR DIET: THE BIGGEST CONTRIBUTORS TO BELLY FAT

You've probably heard that abs are made in the kitchen, not the gym. One client once asked me, "Where is this mythical kitchen that makes abs?" Unfortunately, there are no magic tricks here. We have to do it ourselves, and it starts with knowing what to change and how to change it.

SUGAR

You've probably heard a lot about looking out for added sugar lately, especially now that companies are required to put the amount of added sugars on nutrition labels.

Added sugar means it's not naturally occurring, but added during the processing of the food.

This includes sucrose, dextrose, table sugar, syrups, honey, and sugars from concentrated fruit or vegetable juices.

We're talking sugary drinks, sweet snacks, and desserts. All the good stuff like cookies, brownies, ice cream, doughnuts, etc.

But, too much sugar brings us full circle to belly fat because guess what? When you eat too much sugar, you become more insulin resistant. Remember earlier when I talked about how that contributes to belly fat?

Many of us don't even look at the added sugar on the nutrition label; maybe you didn't even know it was there. But you're going to start doing that now because it will help you make much better choices.

Some foods have naturally occurring sugar like fruit, veggies, dairy products, and grains. Because these have nutritional value, these are foods you should keep in your diet.

It's the added sugar that comes with processed food that's the culprit. It's in our DNA to crave sugar. Remember when you were a kid and all you wanted was candy? Me too.

It's just so yummy, right? But cutting your sugar can make a big difference in losing belly fat.

The American Heart Association recommends the maximum amount of added sugars you should have in a day:

- ✓ For Men: 150 calories per day, which is 37.5 grams or 9 teaspoons
- ✓ For Women: 100 calories per day, which is 25 grams or 6 teaspoons

Getting Rid of Added Sugar
- ✓ **Stop With The Sugary Drinks**—If you drink fruit juice, look for one that's all-natural juice. Get rid of sodas, sugary sports drinks, etc.

And here's something interesting you may not know liquid sugar (like what's in a Coke) is worse than other sugars because your brain doesn't recognize it the same way it does solid calories. Thus, you end up eating more total calories.

✓ **Go For Unsweetened Stuff**—I'm big on yogurt, but once I compared what I was eating (fruity stuff) with plain yogurt I realized just how much added sugar I was eating. The next time you go to the grocery store, give yourself extra time to look at the labels of your staple foods and see if you can swap them out for something with less sugar.

✓ **Eat Whole Foods**—These are foods that haven't been processed, like pretty much any fruit, vegetable, beans, nuts, seafood, meat, etc.

✓ **Watch Your Alcohol**—I am a big fan of wine; consuming some in small increments isn't terrible. But alcohol has a lot of sugar in it. Avoid mixed drinks if you can because those have the most sugar. More on that next.

✓ **Skip Sugary Desserts and Snacks**—If you eat any kind of meal replacement bars, look at the label to see how much sugar is in there. KIND bars are usually a good choice. Just choose one around two hundred calories, at least six grams of protein, three grams of fiber, and no more than six grams of sugar. If you have a sweet tooth, there are many low-carb options if you take the time to look, or make your own. You can usually substitute unsweetened applesauce for sugar in many recipes.

ALCOHOL

For a lot of us, drinking is fun at the end of the day to unwind or in social situations, and in some ways, a little can have health benefits like reducing cardiovascular disease risk if you drink red wine.

But, as I mentioned above, alcohol can have a lot of sugar in it. One glass of wine (five oz) has about 1.2 grams of sugar. A margarita can have up to 12 grams. Here are just some of the things about alcohol that may make you cut down.

✓ **Alcohol is Considered Empty Calories**—Empty calories mean that there's very little nutritional value in many drinks.

✓ **Alcohol Contributes to Belly Fat**—Drinking means extra calories and sugar, so that drink is going right to your belly.

- ✓ **You Make Bad Choices**—Drinking lowers your inhibitions, so you're much more likely to eat the pizza and not care about the consequences.
- ✓ **Alcohol Affects Sleep**—There have been many studies about this and research has shown that alcohol can lead to waking up during the night. Remember that sleep deprivation also contributes to belly fat.

If you drink, monitor how much you're drinking and what you're drinking. There are some great apps out there that help. Drinker's Helper (www.drinkershelper.com) is a great way to track your drinking and set goals to quit or cut down.

UNHEALTHY FATS

You've probably heard about saturated fat and that you should avoid it. If you're trying to lose belly fat, that's exactly what you want to do.

Research shows that if you eat saturated fat, you build more fat and less muscle. Not only that, but it also determines where fat will be stored in the body. Guess where that is? Around the belly and the liver.

Some foods that have a lot of saturated fat include things like beef, pork, butter, full-fat cheese, and milk. You can avoid saturated fat by limiting these foods and choosing more lean protein like chicken, fish, and nuts.

PROCESSED AND ULTRA-PROCESSED FOODS

Some processed foods are good for you like canned fruit in water or bagged spinach. Then you have food that experts call "ultra-processed."

These are foods with preservatives, added sugar, added salt, and other weird ingredients you probably can't pronounce.

One study found that ultra-processed food makes up about 60 percent of calories in the American diet. Oh, dear.

Another study found that people who were given ultra-processed food ate more and gained more weight. There are also connections with obesity, cancer, and high blood pressure, just to name a few.

The thing about ultra-processed food, other than a lot of additives that aren't found in nature, is that the processing can sometimes strip nutrients, fiber, and other important things your body needs.

In the next chapter we'll talk more about this, but for now some of the worst processed foods you can eat include things like sweetened cereal, white bread, flavored potato chips, fried chicken, and granola bars, just to name a few.

You'll learn in the next chapter how to swap these out.

EATING REFINED CARBS INSTEAD OF WHOLE CARBS

When you hear the word *carb*, you might think you can't eat them because they're bad. But carbs include a wide variety of very healthy foods.

But cutting the refined carbs, much like the ultra-processed foods I mentioned before, is your first step in cutting that extra sugar out of your diet. Sugar, bread, candy . . . those are the foods you want to avoid and once you cut those kinds of carbs out, studies show that you lose weight—particularly around the belly—and you have a lower appetite

Whole carbs have some nutritional value, vitamins and minerals, and fiber. Things like quinoa, vegetables, oats, and bananas.

And here's something else to think about: Low-fat foods. If you were around in the '80s, you've probably been part of the low-fat craze. This made us believe that eating fat *makes* us fat.

The problem is, low-fat foods often replace fat with sugar. Eating healthy fats can keep us much more satisfied. You're much better off eating healthy fats like avocados or 4 percent yogurt instead of avoiding full-fat choices.

More on that in the next chapter.

YO-YO DIETING

We've all probably been there at one point or another. Now, what seems counterintuitive is the fact that undereating can sabotage your weight loss goals. When you don't eat enough, your metabolism slows down because your body isn't getting the fuel it needs for everything you're doing.

When I was growing up, my friends and I did crash diets and skipped meals to lose weight, but this can backfire as your body tries to store energy to fuel your body. And a nasty side effect is that, if you lose weight, some of it is muscle. Your body needs food to fuel your body.

The problem is, when you undereat, your brain thinks you have no access to food, so you end up storing more fat for fuel. That means your metabolism slows down.

Eventually, you get hungry and, like most of us, you go back to your old eating habits. Then you gain back the weight you lost, often even more. In a study published in *Evolution, Medicine, and Public Health* researchers found that when food is abundant, meaning when you're not dieting or restricting, you don't store as much fat as when you're dieting.

Another study found that most people who try short-term diets will regain about 30 to 65 percent of that lost weight in one year.

Here's another reason to get out of dieting. The weight you gain back will be more fat than muscle so you'll end up gaining more weight simply because you've lost the metabolically active tissue and added fat that doesn't do much for weight loss.

And, guess what? It means more belly fat. When you gain back that weight, a lot of it comes back as belly fat.

Here's an eye-opener: one study published in *Obesity* found that, for every two pounds you lose, your appetite increases. Your body is actually trying to get you to eat up to or more than one hundred extra calories. Very rude.

The key here is to work on getting out of the diet mindset and understanding that long-term, sustainable goals are built on healthy behaviors instead of restriction, which is exactly what we're talking about in the next chapter.

Chapter 4
Changes You Can Make to Your Diet Right Now

PANTRY CLEAN-OUT

One of the first things to do is set aside some time to go through your pantry and cabinets and get rid of the things that contribute most to weight gain and belly fat.

✓ **Refined Grains**—Bread, rolls, pasta, crackers, rice, etc. All of these things have a lot of added sugar.

✓ **Junk Food**—Chips, cookies, anything with a lot of sugar and not much nutritional value.

✓ **Instant Cereals**—Flavored oatmeal is a good example. It's usually high in sugar. You can make plain oatmeal and add fruit and a little honey to sweeten it.

✓ **Salad Dressing**—Store-bought salad dressing often has saturated fat, a lot of sodium, added sugar, and extra calories. I have a very easy, yummy recipe for homemade salad dressing in the next section.

✓ **Canned Fish Packed in Oil**—Try the version where it's packed in water.

✓ **Packaged Foods**—If sugar is one of the first three ingredients, get rid of it.

✓ **Trans Fat**—If it has trans fat or hydrogenated oil, get rid of it.

FOOD SWAPS

Once you get rid of the stuff that's a little too tempting, now it's time to see what foods you can swap out for healthier choices. This can save tons of calories and you can still enjoy food.

Instead Of This	Try This
Mayonnaise	Mustard
Sandwich Bread	Romaine Lettuce for Wraps
Soda	Seltzer
Juice	Whole Fruit
Potato Chips	Popcorn
Granola	Steel-Cut Oats
Dessert	Dark Chocolate
Pasta	Spiralized Zucchini and Squash
Store-Bought Dressing	Make Your Own

Here's a really simple dressing recipe that will take you about five minutes:

Ginger Lime Dressing

2 tbsp of Coconut Aminos (similar to soy sauce)
1 tbsp of Lime Juice
½ tsp of Ginger (fresh, grated, or minced)

Mix it together and pour over your favorite salad. It makes about two servings, so you can always double it if you want more.

DRINK MORE WATER

Staying fully hydrated can help you lose weight. Research has found that the more hydrated you are, the more efficiently your body works at everything from regular daily tasks to weight loss.

It also helps:

✓ **Suppress Your Appetite**—First, when we feel thirsty we often think we're hungry. Second, drinking a glass of water before meals (and throughout the day) can make you feel full so you eat less.

✓ **Get Your Metabolism Going**—Drinking water isn't going to lead to a ton of weight loss, but one study published in the *Journal of Clinical Endocrinology & Metabolism* found that drinking two cups of water led to an average of a 30 percent increase in metabolism.

- ✓ **Burn Fat**—Your body needs water to do many bodily functions, including burning fat. Dehydration can hinder fat burning, although experts aren't sure why. It may be hormones or the fact that water expands in your cells, which might play a role.
- ✓ **Give You Energy for Exercise and Movement**—Dehydration can make you feel tired and can increase your stress hormones.

Those are just some of the many benefits of staying hydrated. The Mayo Clinic recommends about 15.5 cups (3.7 liters) a day for men and about 11.5 cups (2.7 liters) a day for women.

You may need more if you're exercising, pregnant, in hot weather, or breastfeeding.

You'll know if you're hydrated if you don't feel thirsty and your urine is light yellow or colorless.

One of my favorite things to use at home is a water bottle that shows you when to drink and how much. HydroMATE has a variety of choices and you can find them at Amazon.com (www.amazon.com). It's one of those enormous bottles you might see a gym-goer using, but keeping it on my desk reminds me to drink more frequently.

EAT MORE PROTEIN

Protein is one of the most important nutrients that help you lose belly fat. Experts have found that it can reduce cravings by up to 60 percent (!) and boost your metabolism by about 80 to a 100 calories a day.

It keeps you satisfied so you eat fewer calories. It takes your body more energy to break down protein than carbs or fat and it also helps you avoid weight gain and lose belly fat.

That's quite a bit of bang for your buck. Studies show that older adults, those over 50, often don't get enough protein. And if you're doing the workouts in this book, you'll need more.

One study published in the *Journal of Aging and Physical Activity* suggests older adults who lift weights should have between 1.0 and 1.3 grams per kilogram per day.

To make it easy for you, this calculator at Trifecta can walk you through the process of figuring out just how much protein you need (https:www.trifectanutrition.com/protein-calculator). To keep it simple, try to have some protein at every meal.

GREAT SOURCES OF PROTEIN

Fish

Chicken

Pork tenderloin

Beans

Nuts and seeds

Tofu

Eggs

Yogurt or cottage cheese

Broccoli

CUT OUT ADDED SUGAR

I've been harping on this for the entire book and you already have a lot of ideas for cutting added sugar. The most important tips on this topic include:

- ✓ Read Food Labels for Added Sugar
- ✓ Skip the Juice and Eat Whole Fruits and Veggies
- ✓ Get Rid of Refined Carbs
- ✓ Skip the Soda

Even just doing one of these will immediately cut down your sugar and, listen, the more you work on your sugar, the less you'll crave it.

EAT MORE FIBER

I'm sure you wish I would recommend eating more ice cream and pizza to lose weight because fiber isn't always as sexy.

But, getting enough in your diet can help you lose more belly fat. In one study posted in *Obesity*, researchers looked at lifestyle factors that affected belly fat. Those who ate more soluble fiber and exercised lost the most belly fat.

It's important to know that there are different types of fiber: soluble and insoluble fiber.

You need both but, for belly fat, the soluble kind is what works on that.

A QUICK LOOK AT INSOLUBLE FIBER
Insoluble fiber doesn't mix with water, which is what helps you poop and avoid constipation.

Here are some examples:

Beans
Peas
Whole grains like wheat berries
Fruits and veggies
Wheat bran

These should be a regular part of your diet, but like everything in life, there can always be too much of a good thing.

Too much fiber, which experts suggest is around 70 grams a day, can have negative effects including:

- ✓ Bloating
- ✓ Gas
- ✓ Constipation
- ✓ Cramping and/or diarrhea
- ✓ Decrease in appetite
- ✓ Too much weight loss

If you experience a lot of bloating, start removing some fiber from your diet such as raw vegetables, beans, whole grains, nuts, and seeds.

A QUICK LOOK AT SOLUBLE FIBER
Soluble fiber has a substance that mixes with water which forms a gel-like substance that slows down how fast your stomach releases digested food into your belly.

That sounds gross, but this kind of fiber helps you lose belly fat and prevent gaining more belly fat.

The same study I mentioned before found that people who increased their fiber by 10 grams had a 3.7 percent lower risk of gaining belly fat.

There are other benefits of soluble fiber including better gut health, which also helps you lose belly fat. It helps reduce your appetite by balancing your hunger hormones.

Sounds good, right? So how much fiber do you need? The USDA recommends men eat 30 to 38 grams per day, and women should aim for 20 to 21 grams per day.

GREAT SOURCES OF SOLUBLE FIBER

One cup of black beans has 15 grams of carbs. You're more than halfway there!

Lima beans. I'm not a fan, but you get 5.3 grams per ¾ cup.

Brussels Sprouts—4 grams per cup

Avocados—This may surprise you, but one avocado has 13.5 grams of fiber, which includes both soluble and insoluble. It also has healthy fat, which keeps you full and satisfied.

Sweet Potatoes—4 grams of fiber, 2 of which are insoluble.

Those are just a few ideas. Others include broccoli, pears, turnips, figs, and apricots. Combine a few of these and you'll meet your fiber needs. Remember to take it slow.

EAT HEALTHY FATS

Remember what I said earlier: Fat doesn't make you fat. It's better to eat full-fat foods than low-fat, which usually has added sugar.

BEST HEALTHY FATS

✓ Cooking oils like olive oil, canola oil, or sunflower oil
✓ Avocados
✓ Chia seeds
✓ Dark chocolate (it's not all boring, right?)
✓ Fatty fish like salmon
✓ Flaxseeds

✓ Almonds, walnuts, and other nuts
✓ Nut butters (I like almond butter)
✓ Yogurt
✓ Tofu

MEAL PREP

You can see from the lists I've made throughout the book that getting rid of belly fat has a lot of moving parts and it can get confusing.

That's where meal prepping comes in. What that means is getting your stuff ready for a few meals, or all of them if you're ready to jump into the deep end. You make it, portion it out, and that way you can pull it out whenever you're ready for it.

This saves huge amounts of time and headaches. When I started meal prepping, there was no way I was going to spend a whole Sunday cooking and prepping. I am not a fan of cooking, even though I do it.

I'm going to share the things that help me the most in preparing for my week:

✓ **Make or Buy a Roasted Chicken**—You can do so many things with a whole chicken like making chicken wraps for lunch, adding it to a salad, making white bean chicken chili, etc. I usually buy it, my husband breaks it down, and then I make a list of recipes I can use with it.
✓ **Prep Salads and Veggies**—I really hate making salads, so on Sunday I prep the lettuce (wash it, spin it, wrap it in paper towels, and put it in a baggie), cucumbers, sliced peppers, and dressing. Salads are a great place to add flaxseed or chia seeds. Two birds, one stone.
✓ **Prep Your Snacks**—I keep a mix of my favorite snacks in portions and I always have hummus in the fridge for a quick dip with veggies.
✓ **Double Your Recipes**—I also make twice as much food so I can have it as leftovers the next day.

Other shortcuts you can take if you have to make things easier include buying bagged salad, cut-up fruits, and veggies, and having a backup plan for days when you're too busy or tired to make anything.

Granola bars for snacks frozen meals like Amy's organic meals, or Green Giant Protein Bowls. Avoid too much sodium and, of course, added sugar.

READ FOOD LABELS

I've mentioned things like saturated fat, trans fat, sugar, sodium, and other things to look at in a food label.

I also talked about the fact that changing your eating habits starts with knowing what you're already eating to see if you need to do a food swap.

I have a simple manual that shows you what you should look for in food labels. You can download that here: www.bit.ly/3p8IfBZ.

It gives you a crash course in all the things I've already talked about so you can make better health choices.

You may have to practice this, but it's one of the most important things you can teach yourself to learn how to eat better and lose belly fat.

MIND YOUR PORTION SIZES

- ✓ **Use Smaller Plates**—Sounds silly, but what your eyes see isn't always what your body needs.
- ✓ **Use Portion Control Plates**—If you head over to Amazon, you'll find a wide variety of portion control plates that help you manage your meals. It gives you a very good idea of how much you should eat for each nutrient.
- ✓ **Meal Prep**—I mentioned this above. Portioning out your meals means you always know how much you're eating. I have a system I really love, the 21-Day Portion Control Container Kit from Amazon. It comes with a guide, so you know how to use them to portion out your food.

Remember this: A serving size is not the same as portion size. According to the American Heart Association (AHA), a portion is how much you choose to eat at one time.

A serving size is the amount of food listed on the nutrition label, which could mean multiple portion sizes, if that makes sense. Why are they different?

Because companies can choose their own serving sizes. Plus, we're eating more calories, eating out more (and restaurants often have huge portions), and we have no idea what a portion is many times.

For a visual, visit the blog at healthyeating.org entitled "Mindfulness + Simple Portion Size Tips for Better Eating" and scroll down for a graphic showing you exactly how to get the right portions.

Some quick tips:

One portion of cheese is the size of your index finger
For apples, peaches, cereal carrots, shoot for a fist-sized portion
For pasta and rice, a handful
For protein, like chicken, the size of the palm of your hand

If you work on this, you'll be able to eyeball these.

TRACK YOUR EATING

Finally, we get to another important thing tracking your eating. You don't have to do this forever, but I usually recommend my clients keep a log for a week or so.

When you do this, be patient with yourself and just write what you're already eating and when along with your hunger levels to track your emotional eating.

You can keep it simple, go high-tech, or track as much as you want. Here are some options:

- ✓ **Use Your Own Journal**—Write down what you eat. No need to get fancy, although it does help to measure your portions so you know if you're going overboard.
- ✓ **Use a Ready-Made Journal**—I like the *Hello New Me* journal, available at Amazon for just about eight dollars. You can track both exercise and diet.
- ✓ **Do it Online**—MyFitnessPal is a favorite among my clients, and it's both online or available as an app on your phone.

✓ **Use a Smartphone App**—I mentioned MyFitnessPal, which is free; WW (Weight Watchers), which has a great interactive way to grocery shop and log your foods; and Fooducate, which helps you navigate food labels and keep you smart about your food. These are just a few and you may need to find the one that's easiest for you to use.

Here's a quick tip for logging your food: Take a picture of each meal, and then you can log it when you get time.

Sometimes, if you don't log it right away, you forget what you ate. You may forget those extra snacks or chips.

I know I like to forget those, too.

Chapter 5
Let's Talk about Exercise

CARDIO FOR LOSING BELLY FAT

I know, I know, exercise can be a challenge for many of us and, as I mentioned previously, a lot of us find it hard to exercise because we're tired, may have injuries or other health conditions, and may find it hard to know where to get started.

But, if you want to feel strong, independent, and lose belly fat, it's more of a necessity rather than a luxury.

There are three things you'll work on in this book: Cardio, strength training, and flexibility. Mixed in with that will be mobility and balance, and all of these things will make you look and feel better.

GENERAL EXERCISE GUIDELINES

The general guidelines for older adults according to the *Journal of the American Medical Association* include:

One hundred fifty to three hundred minutes of moderate activity a week. This works out to about 30 minutes five days a week or 60 minutes five days a week. Or you can do 75 or more minutes of vigorous-intensity exercise.

You can also mix and match. I'll give you some suggested schedules so you can pick what works for you.

Keep in mind that you should start where you are, which may mean 10 to 20 minutes a few times a week, and slowly work your way up.

Now on to the different intensities and how you can monitor them.

What is Moderate-Intensity Exercise?

Moderate-intensity exercise means that, whatever you're doing, you should be able to carry on a conversation without gasping for air.

So, things like:

- ✓ Brisk walking
- ✓ Swimming
- ✓ Low-impact aerobics
- ✓ Dancing
- ✓ Vigorous yard work
- ✓ Cycling

Moderate-intensity exercise is about 64 to 76 percent of your maximum heart rate. I'll show you how to measure that down the road.

What is Vigorous-Intensity Exercise?

This intensity is just what it sounds like. You will definitely know you're exercising at this level. You can talk, but only in short bursts before you lose your breath.

This is about 77 to 93 percent of your maximum heart rate.

Some ideas include:

- ✓ Running
- ✓ High-impact aerobics
- ✓ Sports—tennis, basketball, etc.
- ✓ Fast cycling
- ✓ Plyometric training
- ✓ Hiking
- ✓ Speed walking

Monitoring Your Intensity

What we're talking about is your target heart rate zone, which includes the zones to work in to make your workouts effective and efficient. These numbers are expressed in percentages. If you want to go that route, it's about calculating a range to work within your most effective heart rate zone to reach your goals.

There are formulas out there to guide you through the process of finding your target heart rate zones, but I like using an online calculator like the one at Acefitness.org.

The article walks you through a step-by-step process of how to calculate your target heart rate zones, along with your maximum heart rate and resting heart rate, both of which are a part of the formula.

However, you don't need to get fancy to figure out how hard you're working. It can be as easy as using a Rate of Perceived Exertion (RPE) chart.

So, what is RPE? You use a scale of 1 to 10 to assess how you feel based on your exertion. For example, if you're sitting around, that would be a 1 on the scale. If you're sprinting, that would be closer to a 9 or 10.

Your RPE is not based on how fast you're walking or moving. It's based solely on how you feel during the exercise.

This is a subjective measurement. You could take a brisk walk and maybe it feels like a level 5, while someone else might rate it as a 6 or 7.

The most used RPE scale is the Borg Rating of Perceived Exertion, which gives you a scale from 6 to 20.

Many of my clients find this confusing, so I have an easier version that I use with my clients.

This RPE Scale gives you an idea of how hard you're working on a scale of 1 to 10.

Sample Rate of Perceived Exertion Scale
Level 1—I'm lying on the couch watching Netflix
Level 2—I'm puttering around the house
Level 3—I'm doing something more energetic, like household chores
Level 4—I'm taking a stroll or some other activity that's starting to feel harder
Level 5—I'm definitely exercising now and am breathing harder
Level 6—I'm breathing harder and I'm starting to have trouble talking
Level 7—I'm working even harder and I'm feeling it
Level 8—I'm breathing even harder and talking is not going to happen
Level 9—I'm working hard and don't know if I can keep going
Level 10—I can't talk, I'm gasping, and have no idea why I'm doing this to myself

If you use some kind of activity tracker or heart rate monitor (I like using my Apple Watch), you can use the RPE scale and check in on your heart rate at different levels of intensity. For example, when I walk, it feels around a 5 on the RPE scale and my heart rate might be around 125 or 130 beats per minute. That gives me a reference point to compare other exercises and how they affect my heart rate.

You'll learn more about your body and what heart rate matches how you're feeling.

THE BEST CARDIO FOR LOSING BELLY FAT

The best cardio for losing belly fat is pretty much any cardio you'll do. It really is a matter of doing some kind of rhythmic motions that gets your heart rate up. Even vigorously raking leaves can count.

This is especially true if you haven't been doing much cardio. Any movement you add is going to benefit you tremendously. However, there are a couple of types of cardio you might want to consider.

We'll start with high-intensity interval training.

HIGH-INTENSITY INTERVAL TRAINING (HIIT)

Don't let the name scare you because you don't have to do things like sprints or jumps to get a good HIIT workout.

What HIIT means is doing short periods of intense exercise followed by a short rest period and then repeating that process. But, how intense that exercise is depends on you.

If you're a beginner, you'll find that many movements will feel intense. If you're a regular, you might need to up the ante for more challenging exercises.

The first few weeks of this program are where you'll figure out what feels intense to you, and I'll give you some guidance on that.

Here's an example: You go out for a walk and every minute or so you speed up so you're walking as fast as you can, like you're trying to catch a bus that's about to leave.

Your heart rate increases, you're breathing a little heavier, but you know you get to slow down soon.

You can choose something in the distance to walk to (this is called Fartlek training), you can time it, or you can use an app on your smartphone.

The point is you alternate something harder with something easier for the duration of your workout. Think of it as doing rounds of exercises. You get your heart rate up with a challenging exercise and then bring it down with a less challenging exercise.

Examples of HIIT Workouts
- ✓ Walking—Alternating regular walking with short bursts of speeding up
- ✓ On a treadmill—Walking at a steady pace for a period of time (say, 40 seconds to 1 minute) and then either speeding up or raising the incline for either the same amount of time or, for beginners, less time (say, 20 to 30 seconds).
- ✓ At-home exercise—Marching in place, then either speeding it up, walking up and down a staircase, or walking around your house at a faster pace.

The Benefits of HIIT
- ✓ **It helps you lose belly fat**. One study published in the *Journal of the American Geriatrics Society*, researchers took participants with belly fat through 10 weeks of HIIT, starting slowly and increasing intensity over the course of several weeks. They concluded that 10 weeks of vigorous intensity interval training improved body composition in older adults with belly fat.
- ✓ **Improves cardio health and muscle strength**
- ✓ **Improves overall health**
- ✓ **More fatburning and weight loss** than some other types of training
- ✓ **HIIT workouts are usually short**, around 10 to 20 minutes depending on where you start out
- ✓ **You only have to do them a couple of times a week** because your body needs recovery time

Sample Home HIIT Workout for Beginners
Below is a sample home workout that includes a variety of low-impact exercises, although you can adapt the workout to your fitness level.

The Workout: HIIT
Equipment: One dumbbell or medicine ball (4-8 lbs), a towel, and a chair

Tip: Warm up with a few minutes of light cardio or try the Warm-up Workout later in this book. You want to slowly raise your heart rate and get the circulation going before you do anything too strenuous.

How it Works: Do each exercise for the suggested time (or what you can do), one after the other. Rest if you need to between exercises and complete 1 to 3 circuits. That means going through all the exercises once and then again if you have the energy. You may need to work up to more circuits, so don't worry if one is enough for now.

How to Modify: To change the intensity of each exercise, you can:

- ✓ Add bigger arm movements—This will push your heart rate up higher
- ✓ Increase your range of motion—The bigger the movements, the more intense the exercise will feel
- ✓ Add more impact—The exercises in this workout are low impact, but if you want more intensity, you can add jumps to many of the exercises
- ✓ Be sure to skip any moves that cause any pain or discomfort
- ✓ Similarly, you can cut out the arms, have a smaller range of motion, and keep things low-impact for a lower intensity.

SQUAT WITH CRESCENT KNEES

Step out to the right into a squat, sending the hips back and keeping the abs in. As you stand, bring the right knee up and make a circle with your knee towards the right wall, opening the hips. Repeat for 30 seconds and switch to the other side.

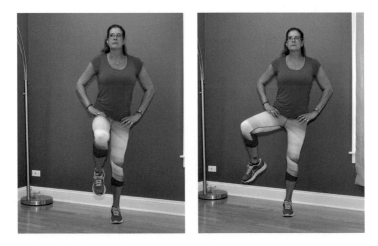

STEP OUTS WITH OVERHEAD REACH

Keep the weight on the right leg and step out with the left foot. Take the left arm up at a diagonal as you step out. Step the foot back in, lower the arm and repeat for 30 seconds before switching sides.

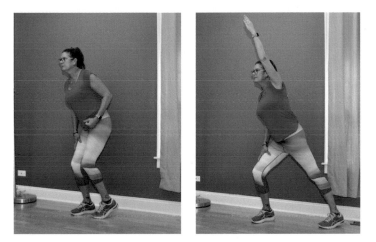

KNEE SMASH

With the weight on the right leg and arms straight up at a diagonal, pull the left knee up towards the chest while bringing the arms down and squeezing the abs. Repeat as fast as you can for 30 seconds and switch sides. You can add a jump if you want a higher intensity.

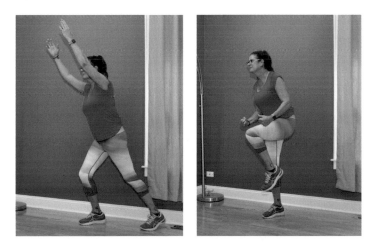

SQUAT WITH KNEE LIFT

With the feet about hip-width apart, squat, sending the hips back. Press through the heels to stand as you bring the right knee up and the arms overhead. Lower and repeat either on the same leg (holding on to a chair or the wall for balance if needed), or alternate sides for 30 seconds.

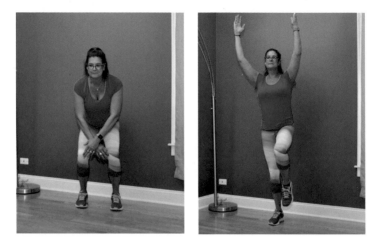

HEEL DIGS

Start with the feet together and take the left leg forward, placing the heel on the floor and pushing the hands down. Jump or step to the right, like you're stepping or jumping over a ball and bring the right heel forward, arms down. Alternate heel digs on each side for 30 seconds.

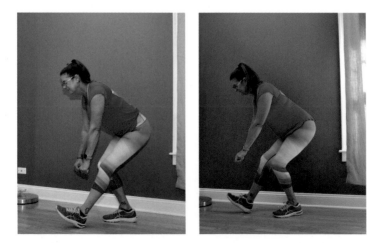

CROSSOVER KNEE SMASH

With the hands behind the head, bring the left knee across the body while bringing the right elbow towards the knee, squeezing the core. Go as fast as you can for 30 seconds before switching sides.

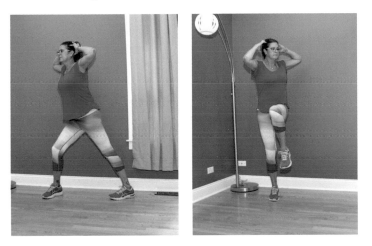

PUDDLEJUMPER WITH LIFTS

Take a low, wide step out to the right like you're stepping over a large puddle. Step the feet together and lift up on the toes while taking the arms straight up. You can also add a jump for more intensity. Repeat, going from side to side for 30 seconds.

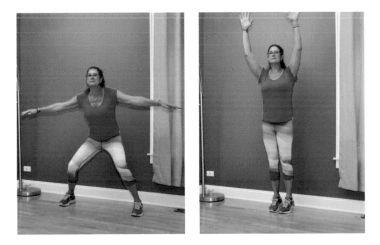

SIDE SQUAT SCOOP

Step out to the right into a squat while scooping the arms in front of your body. Step back and repeat to the other side, squatting and scooping the arms. Repeat for 30 seconds.

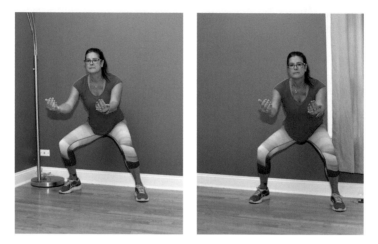

DUMBBELL SWING

Hold a dumbbell or medicine ball (4-10 lbs) with feet hip-width apart. Squat, and swing the dumbbell between the legs. Power through the hips to take the weight overhead. Repeat for 30 seconds.

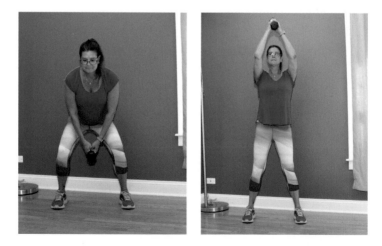

LOW-IMPACT JUMPING JACK

Step out to the left touching the toe to the floor while taking the arms up at a diagonal. Circle the arms the other way as you turn in the opposite direction and step to the right. Alternate sides as quickly as you can while moving the arms like you're making a circle with them. Repeat for 30 seconds. For more intensity, do regular jumping jacks.

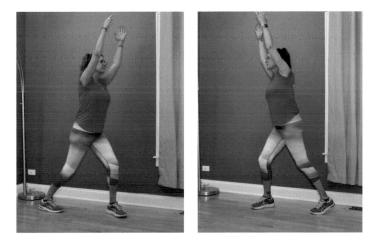

SIDE TO SIDE PUNCH

Turn to the right, stepping the left foot out to the side while punching towards the right with the left arm. Step back and repeat on the other side, lunging to the left and punching with the right hand. Repeat for 30 seconds.

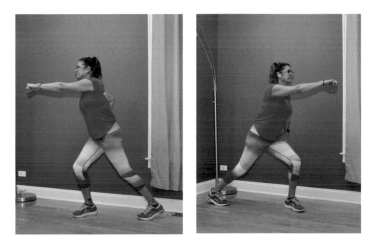

CURTSY LUNGES

Start with the feet wide and lower into a squat. Now take the right foot back and at a diagonal behind the left foot as in a curtsy. Step the right foot back and move as quickly as you can for 30 seconds before switching sides.

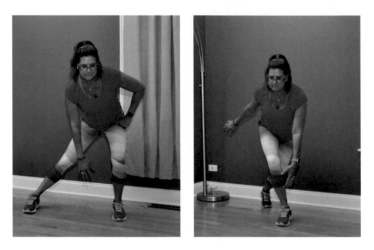

REAR TOWEL SLIDES

Hold on to a chair for balance if needed and place a towel under the left foot. Bend the left knee and slide the right foot back and in as fast as you can. Repeat for 30 seconds and then switch sides.

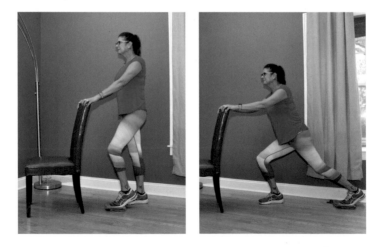

SIDE TOWEL SLIDES

Hold on to a chair for balance if you need to. Place a towel under the left foot. Slide the left foot straight out to the side and then back in as quickly as you can. Repeat for 30 seconds and switch sides.

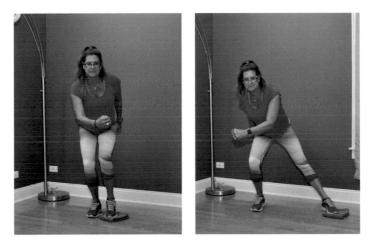

LOW-IMPACT STEADY STATE TRAINING (LISS)

On the other side of HIIT is LISS, yet another acronym because fitness experts require them.

Don't worry about understanding all this. Think of it this way: A HIIT workout is short, and involves intervals of higher intensity and recovery.

LISS is the opposite where you work for longer periods of time at a low, more comfortable intensity. This is how I usually introduce my new clients or those who haven't been exercising lately, to build endurance and body strength so you can add more variety.

Steady-state training means a heart rate around 50 to 65 percent of your maximum heart rate or about a Level 4 or 5 on the RPE scale. One study showed that training at a lower intensity can burn more fat.

The downside is that it does increase your training time. Experts usually recommend about 45-minute steady state sessions but, of course, you should always start out with what feels good to you and gradually work your way up.

The Benefits of LISS Training

✓ Improves your body's ability to use fat, instead of carbs as fuel. It also improves fat distribution.

- ✓ It's great for all fitness levels. Because it's easier to do and more gentle on the body, people are often more comfortable starting with this type of training.
- ✓ Your body recovers more easily because you're putting less stress on your heart and body.
- ✓ LISS is also great for training for endurance events as well as recovering after challenging workouts.

Examples of LISS
- ✓ Cycling
- ✓ Brisk walking or jogging
- ✓ Swimming
- ✓ Cardio machines like the treadmill or the elliptical

If you're just starting out, this is a sample cardio schedule I might make for you:

Day 1	Day 2	Day 3	Day 4	Day 5	Day 6	Day 7
	LISS (10–20 Min)	Rest	HIIT (10–15 Min)	Rest		LISS (10–20 Min)

Later, I'll provide a full sample schedule that includes both cardio and your resistance training workouts.

STRENGTH TRAINING FOR LOSING BELLY FAT

GENERAL STRENGTH TRAINING GUIDELINES FOR SENIORS
The Centers for Disease Control recommend the following:
- ✓ Lift weights two non-consecutive days a week
- ✓ Choose at least one exercise per muscle group. That would include:
  - » Chest: pushups, chest press, chest fly
  - » Back: one-arm row, reverse fly, back extensions
  - » Shoulders: overhead press, lateral raises, front raises
  - » Biceps: biceps curls, concentration curls, hammer curls

- » Triceps: triceps extensions, kickbacks, skull crushers
- » Lower body: squats, lunges, deadlifts
- » Core: bird dog, modified plank, bridge, bicycle
- ✓ Perform at least one set of 8-12 reps of each exercise. An example of a repetition is doing one biceps curl. If you do 12 biceps curls, that's a set. As you get stronger, you should add more sets, usually up to three sets.
- ✓ Lift as much weight as you can for the number of reps you're doing. For example, if you do 12 biceps curls and you feel like you could do more than another 4 or 5 reps, you may need to increase your weight. More about that in the following chapters.

How to Choose Your Weight

This is where things can get tricky and many people worry that they're not lifting enough or they're lifting too much.

In gym and bodybuilding settings, they determine how much weight a person lifts by using a one-rep Max. This is the maximal weight a person can lift for only one rep with the correct form and technique.

They would then take a percentage of that weight that matches the number of reps they want to do.

Way complicated and not safe for most of us.

The best way for us to determine how much weight to use is to guess. Yep, it's a guessing game and the only way you can get it wrong is if you wake up the next day after weight training and you can't move because you're very sore. We'll talk about that.

In choosing your weight, consider the following:
- ✓ Your larger muscle groups can handle more weight: your legs, glutes, chest, and back
- ✓ Smaller muscles need less weight: calves, biceps, triceps, and shoulders

There's more to this, but I'll be making suggestions in every workout for the amount of weight to use for each exercise. Your job is to do the following:

1. Pick a weight from the suggested range for the exercise

2. Pay close attention to your body—if you can't get halfway through the set, lighten up. If you could go on forever, add more weight.
3. Keep in mind that it may take you a few workouts before you know what works. It's okay to switch weights when you need to.
4. If you're a beginner, any weight will make you stronger.
5. Err on the side of caution to avoid soreness and injury
6. Also keep in mind that every day is different. Some days you can lift more and some days you need to pull back. That's normal!

Delayed Onset of Muscle Soreness (DOMS)

If you've ever exercised or done something new like, say, shoveling snow for the first time in months, you know what DOMS is. You wake up the next day and feel muscles you never knew you had.

DOMS usually happens when you're starting a new workout or making changes, like adding exercises, weight, reps, or sets later in the program.

It's normal to feel stiff and sore after a new workout. You may experience:

- ✓ Dull, diffuse pain and tenderness
- ✓ Stiffness
- ✓ Swelling
- ✓ Decreased strength of the exercised muscle
- ✓ Wincing every time you sit down or stand up

This can happen 1 to 3 days after your workout. One note—if you can barely move, you know you overdid it and should take an extra rest day and/or pull back on your next workout.

How to Deal with DOMS

When you have post-workout soreness, it's mostly a waiting game. However, there are some things than can help temporarily:

- ✓ NSAIDs like Advil or other over-the-counter anti-inflammatories. Be sure to check with your doctor if you're on other medication
- ✓ Massage

- ✓ Cold packs
- ✓ Exercise or movement—This gets the blood circulation going so you feel better, but the effect is usually just temporary

As I mentioned before, it's better to err on the side of caution with the weights. If it's too easy, you'll know and can then make changes to your next workout.

Discomfort vs. Pain

Anytime you do something physical, there will probably be a level of discomfort. What we want to do is distinguish between normal discomfort that comes from exertion and actual pain. Whenever you start anything new, you'll experience discomfort. But feeling pain is very different and should be a red flag.

You should see your doctor and stop exercising if you experience any of the following:

- ✓ Sharp, shooting pain in any of your joints during workouts or when resting
- ✓ Any pain that lasts more than a week or two
- ✓ If you feel a strained or pull muscle. Sometimes this can be a mild injury that heals overnight, or something that requires R.I.C.E.—rest, ice, compression, and elevation. You may want to see your doctor if it goes on for more than a day or two

Sometimes stopping is the best idea. You always have another day, right? And if the pain persists, be sure to call your doc.

Rewarding Yourself

Too often, we forget about this part, especially as we get older. We forget that we deserve to celebrate our successes, even if they're things we "should" be doing anyway.

Studies have shown that rewarding ourselves can increase our activity levels. Part of how we consistently workout has to do with building a habit so that it becomes second nature to get up, put on our workout clothes, and get moving.

Creating the habit is the tough part, and any good exercise program should include regular rewards to keep you motivated and to celebrate your success.

The more you reinforce the habit of working out, the more likely you're going to do it instead of skip it.

So, let's talk about a way to reward yourself for exercise. There are a lot of different ways to set up a reward system and they involve different levels. You should use all three!

- ✓ **Immediate rewards**—This kind of reward satisfies our need for instant gratification. This can be time built into your actual workout where you spend some time doing something you enjoy. The only catch here is that you probably don't want to use food as a reward, although having some of your favorite foods is not a bad thing as long as you don't overdo it. One thing I do to reward myself is watching a favorite show on Netflix while I'm working out. Another client of mine likes to mess around on her iPad while she walks on the treadmill. As long as you're paying attention, think of something you'd enjoy and you'll be much more likely to stick to your workouts.
- ✓ **Regularly Scheduled Rewards**—One trick I've used to keep myself on track is to reward myself at the end of a week of workouts. How many workout clothes did I sweat through? And how can I make my husband wash them if he, in fact, knows where the washing machine is? This reward can be as simple as taking time to read a book, take a bath, get a pedicure, listen to music, putter in the yard, or hang out with friends with a glass of wine.
- ✓ **Long-Term Rewards**—These are great because you have something to look forward to. This could be a monthly reward for staying on track as much as you can. You could plan a vacation, a weekend getaway, a night out, a massage, or any other activities you enjoy but probably don't get to do that often. Plan something. Put it in your calendar. Make reservations. Commit to pampering yourself. It makes it all worthwhile.

BEST STRENGTH TRAINING FOR LOSING BELLY FAT

Now to the nitty gritty of what we'll be doing in the next few weeks. The road I'm taking you on includes one of the best ways to lose belly fat: circuit training.

You'll learn more about what circuit training is throughout the rest of this book, but know that this is a great way to burn more calories and lose fat. This is because your body actually burns more calories after your workout to help your body get back to its usual state before exercise.

Circuit training can have many definitions. It can be all strength training, all cardio, or a mix of them together. We're going to focus on where we get the most bang for our buck, which is with circuit training combined with compound movements.

Keep on reading to find out just how effective this training protocol can be.

WHAT ARE COMPOUND EXERCISES?

Compound exercises are moves that involve multiple muscles and joints. Think of a squat. That involves your hips, knees, and calves, as well as your quads, hamstrings, and core. Now think of a biceps curl, which involves curling a weight up and down.

That only uses one muscle group and one joint action, also known as isolation exercises. Both of these exercises are important for strength and fitness, but if you want to lose fat and build muscle, compound exercises are a great choice.

For example, in the total body strength circuit workouts, you'll see a variety of compound exercises like squats with an overhead press, lunges with a lateral raise, and rear lunges with a row. All of these help build more muscle, strength, balance, and flexibility.

The Benefits of Doing Compound Exercises

- ✓ **You burn more calories**—The more muscles you work, the more you burn, especially if you combine a lower body exercise with an upper body exercise. The largest muscles in your body are your glutes, so involving them along with your arms or shoulders means you automatically burn more calories.
- ✓ **Better balance and coordination**—One thing we want to work on with this program is being strong, fit, and staying independent. The more compound exercises you do, the more coordinated and stronger you'll be.
- ✓ **Better flexibility**—While we often think of static stretching to improve flexibility, compound exercises are a dynamic way to increase flexibility. As you're moving your joints through a full range of motion, whenever

you can, you're also lengthening the surrounding tissues which will only improve your flexibility, something we need to protect as we get older.

✓ **You build more muscle**—Compound exercises involve more muscle groups, which means you can lift more weight than you would with more isolation exercises. That's going to increase your muscle mass, which in turn will help you shed fat and improve your body composition.

✓ **An elevated heart rat**e—Compound exercises not only build strength, but they often raise your heart rate as much as a cardio workout could. It's this intensity that allows you to have the best of both worlds: cardio and strength in the same workout with multiple physical and health benefits.

WHAT IS CIRCUIT TRAINING?

Okay, so we know all about compound exercises and the benefits they provide. Let's bring in the circuit training part of the equation, which only increases your chances of losing fat, gaining muscle, and being strong.

Circuit training is a kind of metabolic training that uses unique movements, like the compound exercises I just talked about, to increase your metabolism so you lose more body fat.

Circuit training is a protocol which involves going from one exercise to the next with little or no rest. This does some amazing things for your body and mind, a workout that combines all the things we want to work on, like endurance and strength.

Here's how this works:

✓ **Rotating through a variety of exercises**: you'll rotate through about 8 to 12 exercises with little or no rest to keep your heart rate up. This type of workout is designed to keep your heart rate elevated.

✓ **Reps and time**: Some exercises will involve doing a certain number of reps, while others will be time-based, usually around 30 seconds of an exercise. If you have a smartphone, there's usually a timer included. There are also a variety of timer apps that offer more options, if you want to set different intervals in the same workout, for example.

✓ **Keep it moving**: With circuit training, the idea is to move through the exercises with minimal rest. But, it's okay to rest in between exercises if your heart rate is high or you feel too breathless. Your endurance will improve the more you practice. Just keep moving around instead of just stopping.

✓ **Short workouts**: Most of the workouts should be between about 20 and 45 minutes, although it may take longer as you learn the exercises and practice your form. The workouts will get longer as the weeks go on, but we'll start you out at a beginner pace so you can get used to it. It's okay if you don't make it all the way through the workouts at first. Just do as much as you can.

✓ **Take time**: These exercises and workouts may be completely new to you. Give yourself permission to take as much time as you need to learn how to do each exercise. There's no time limit! Having good form is more important than how much weight you lift. Good form is different for different exercises, but generally involves good posture, avoiding rounding the shoulders, and keeping your knees in line with the toes when doing standing exercises.

THE BENEFITS OF CIRCUIT TRAINING

Circuit training, like the compound movements we're adding to the mix, have similar benefits and more such as:

✓ Builds more muscle
✓ Improves your heart functionality
✓ Gives you a full body workout
✓ Saves time
✓ Helps you lose weight
✓ Keeps you motivated

These workouts work because they're higher in intensity, involve your entire body, and you get a bonus. Because we're focusing on compound movements, which work more than one muscle group at a time, here are the two things I want you to focus on with circuit training and compound movements:

1. **You burn more calories during the workout**—Every muscle group you involve elevates your heart rate and burns more calories. As you

get stronger and lift heavier weights, you'll get even more bang for your buck because your body becomes much more efficient delivering and extracting oxygen, which helps your cells burn more fat.

2. **You get more afterburn**—You've probably heard of afterburn, but what does it actually mean? In technical terms, this is called EPOC, exercise post-oxygen consumption. This refers to the calories you burn recovering from exercise. The more muscles you work and the more intense the workout, the greater the afterburn.

Chapter 6
The Program

AN OVERVIEW

This 12-week program is designed to target multiple elements of fitness including strength, endurance, balance, core strength, and flexibility. That sounds like a lot, but the workouts are designed to include exercises that target all of these elements, with a focus on losing belly fat.

You'll start out with a foundational workout for the first two weeks and, every two weeks after that, we'll increase the intensity. This allows you to gradually build strength and endurance in a healthy way to avoid injury and too much soreness.

THE BREAKDOWN OF YOUR WORKOUTS

- ✓ **Warm-up**—This includes dynamic moves to help your body get ready for your workouts. The warm-up is a very important part of your workout and you shouldn't skip it. This is how you get your body ready for exercise and avoid injury.
- ✓ **Total body strength circuit workouts**—These workouts include compound exercises, meaning you'll be working multiple muscle groups with a variety of equipment. These workouts will change every two weeks so you have time to perfect the exercises and mix things up so you can continue to challenge your body.
- ✓ **Flexibility workout**—This workout has simple, effective stretches you can do after your workout to cool down and relax. Feel free to do this workout anytime you like, either after working out or just during the day.

- ✓ **Core workout**—There are core moves in each circuit workout, but there's an extra core workout solely focused on your abs and lower back. You'll see a schedule for each series of workouts, but feel free to do the core workout more often. Just wait at least a day in between workouts.
- ✓ **Suggested workout schedule**—For each two weeks, I'll give you a suggested schedule of when to do your strength training, cardio, core, and flexibility workouts. There may be some soreness and discomfort as you change workouts, so allow room for that and give yourself permission to do what you need to do. You can even stay with the same workouts for longer than two weeks to feel more comfortable.

SHOULD YOU SEE YOUR DOCTOR BEFORE YOU GET STARTED?

Before you get started with any new exercise routine, it's a great idea to see your doctor to make sure everything is in working order and you're cleared for exercise.

Oftentimes, we will skip our yearly physicals, so it's a good idea to get one before you start exercising.

You'll definitely want to see your doctor under these circumstances:

- ✓ **You have any pain or injuries**—You don't want to exacerbate any current or older injuries. And it's important to note that pain, which is different from discomfort, should not be part of any workout. The point is, if you do have any pain or injuries, your doctor may have some suggestions about the right exercise for you and/or what you should avoid.
- ✓ **You have any chronic conditions**—If you have heart disease, arthritis, high blood pressure, kidney disease, diabetes, or are being treated for cancer you should check with your doctor for appropriate activities. In many circumstances, exercise is helpful for many of these conditions, but you should get clearance before starting anything you haven't done in a while.
- ✓ **You're on certain medications**—Beta-blockers and calcium channel blockers can change your heart rate response to exercise and may affect

you during a workout. If you're taking a diuretic, this can affect your hydration levels. Check with your doctor to find out what you need to know before you exercise.

✓ **If you ever feel dizzy or unbalanced**—If you've felt these symptoms in the past month or so, you might want to see your doctor before you exercise. You don't want this to happen in the middle of a workout, as it can cause an injury.

When in doubt, make the appointment. It's always good to know what's going on underneath that skin.

WHAT YOU NEED FOR YOUR WORKOUTS

The workouts involve using a variety of equipment, but they start off with more bodyweight exercises and gradually introduce you to tools you can use to increase your strength, fitness, and weight loss.

It may look like a long list but, keep in mind, you don't need to get everything if you don't already have it. I'll have some alternatives to store bought equipment so, if you're budget-conscious, you have some other options.

EQUIPMENT

✓ **Dumbbells**—It's great to have a range of weights, from 3 to about 12 pounds for women, and 5 to 25 for men. If you don't have weights, I recommend starting with three sets of weights—a light set (3 to 5 pounds), a medium set (5 to 8 pounds), and a heavy set (8 to 12 pounds). You can find these at any sporting goods store and, if you're on a budget, check out Play it Again Sports, where you might find some deals.

» **Alternatives to weights**—Other ways to make your own weights include putting change or sand inside a sock or a tennis ball can. You can also use full water bottles or even soup cans for added intensity. Don't be afraid to be creative, yet careful.

✓ **Resistance Bands**—We'll also be using resistance bands for a variety of exercises. I recommend getting a variety because they come in different strengths, they're inexpensive, and they don't take up much room. My favorite bands are made by Spri and you can find their options at Amazon. I would recommend getting yellow, which is a light resistance; green, which is medium; and red, which is a bit harder. Like weights, the tension of the bands corresponds to the exercise so there is a learning curve there to find out the right amount of tension for the exercise.

✓ **Towel**—You'll need a medium-sized towel for a few exercises throughout the program. You'll use it for some sliding exercises and for isolation exercises to involve more muscle groups and an element of balance and coordination.

✓ **Mat**—You'll also want a mat for floor exercises. You're welcome to use a towel if that works better for you. If you have hardwood floors you might want a thicker mat to protect your joints. If you're on carpet, a lighter mat might be a better choice. My favorite is by Yoga Design Lab. It's more expensive so, if you're on a budget, feel free to look at Walmart, Target, or other discount stores.

✓ **A step**—The last two weeks of the program includes a step, but it's completely optional if you don't have one. It's actually a great addition to any home gym because you can use it as a weight bench, for core work, and for cardio. The step consists of a platform that's about four inches high. You can also get risers that go underneath to increase the height (usually by two inches per riser). If you decide to use one, start with just the platform and go from there. I recommend the Original Step, which you can find at sporting goods stores or online.

✓ **An exercise ball**—There are some exercises towards the end of the program that include an exercise ball, which is an excellent way to work on your balance and core strength. My favorite comes from Spri as well as the resistance bands. These exercise balls are high-quality and anti-burst. Just make sure you get the right size for your height. You want to be able to sit on the ball so that your knees are in line with the hips:

Exercise Ball Diameter	Height
45 cm	5' Tall and Under
55 cm	5'1"–5'8"
65 cm	5'9"–6'2"
75 cm	6'3"–6'7"

WORKOUT SHOES

The shoes you wear are very important in your workouts. The right shoes give you a strong foundation to build from, so if you're going to spend money on something, I would recommend spending it on shoes.

Here's where to start:

- ✓ **Go to a Specialty Store**—The people at running and walking stores are able to make recommendations based on your feet and activity. Speciality stores have people who know just what shoes would work for your chosen activity, if that's an option for you.
- ✓ **Choose Shoes to Match Your Activity**—If you're walking or running, make sure you get a shoe specific to that activity. These shoes are made to provide support and cushioning for higher impact activities. I find that running shoes are great for a variety of activities.
- ✓ **Try Cross-trainers**—These are a good all-around choice if you're lifting weights and/or doing cardio at home. Ryka is one of my favorite companies for women and Nike has some great options for everyone.

Your workout shoes should feel comfortable as soon as you put them on. Be sure to wear the workout socks you plan to use so you get the full experience.

WORKOUT CLOTHES

You don't have to wear anything special to exercise, but there are some options that make it more comfortable:

- ✓ Choose loose-fitting clothes like shorts or leggings, and a T-shirt.

✓ Go for sweat-wicking clothes—Cotton isn't great for a sweaty workout. It makes cotton clothing wet and heavy. You can find sweat-wicking clothes (like those made of polyester) anywhere from Walmart or other discount stores to sporting goods stores.

✓ Choose what works for you. There are so many options out there, but you have your style and preferences. Go for what feels good to you. Once you get a sense of the workouts and how your body responds, you'll be able to make better choices about what to wear. If you're working out at home, who cares if your clothes match, right?

ACTIVITY TRACKER (OPTIONAL)

There are so many different activity trackers out there, you could spend a lot of time researching them. If you're not into activity trackers, no problem. You don't have to use one if you don't want to.

For other people, they might want to track a variety of things during their workouts to stay motivated and see how they're improving after starting exercise.

For me, activity trackers are a great option because you learn more about your body—how much activity you get, your general heart rate, and how different exercise activities feel to your body.

Here are a few of the trackers to consider:

✓ **Apple Watch**—This is my personal favorite because it tracks steps, heart rate, workout information (time, calories burned, etc.), and it even lets you know when you've been sitting too long or prompts you to take a minute to breathe. It can be expensive, so consider your budget. The great thing is that these watches can last a long time.

✓ **FitBit**—FitBit has a wide variety of choices for tracking your workouts. There are less expensive versions that track your heart rate and steps, or more expensive versions that include GPS tracking and even oxygen levels.

✓ **Polar**—This company has so many options, you can be someone who just wants to track your heart rate or someone who wants to run a triathlon and track his or her lap splits. Visit their website to compare a variety of heart rate monitors and activity trackers.

SCHEDULING YOUR WORKOUTS

Sometimes it gets confusing when you're trying to schedule a workout program. I'll provide some suggested schedules, but it helps to know how to set up a routine that gets your results, but also gives you the rest you need to recover and get stronger.

Here are some things to consider about scheduling your workouts:

- ✓ **Cardio can usually be done every day**—The only exception to this is if you're doing high-intensity interval training. You usually want to rest at least a day, if not more, before your next HIIT workout. The schedule I provide, which changes for every workout series, includes ideas of when to do HIIT workouts and LISS workouts—remember, those are longer, steady state workouts. Keep in mind that too many HIIT workouts can be added stress on the body, so I like to keep them at twice a week.
- ✓ **Don't work the same muscle groups two days in a row**—The workouts I provide are total body, which means you need at least one day of rest between workouts. This allows your muscles to grow stronger. In fact, the rest days are exactly when your muscles grow the most.
- ✓ **Take rest days as needed**—If you're very sore or tired, you don't have to rely on the suggested schedule I have for you. Take extra rest days as you need to or do a flexibility or core workout in place of other workouts.

Chapter 7
Warm-Up, Core, Cooldown, and Flexibility Workouts

Warming up is one of the most important parts of your workout. Warming up brings your temperature up, which makes your workout more comfortable. The increase in the temperature of your muscles and connective tissue protects you from soft tissue injuries while also allowing your cardiovascular system to adjust blood flow to give your body the oxygen it needs for exercise.

Your warm-up can be anything from walking, cycling, or any other cardio activity that gets your heart rate up.

The exercises below include moves you can do right in your own living room with no equipment needed. Go through the exercises and, if you need more time to warm up, you can repeat them. Plan at least five minutes to warm up.

WARM-UP WORKOUT

The Workout: Warm-up
Equipment: None
How it Works: Do each exercise one after the other and complete 1 to 3 circuits depending on how warmed up you feel. The idea is to get your joints lubricated and your heart rate up for your workout.

STEP TOUCH

Step out to the right side as far as you can, bringing the arms up and out to shoulder level. Bring the left foot next to the right, touch the floor, and then step back to the left, repeating the move while alternating sides for 30 seconds.

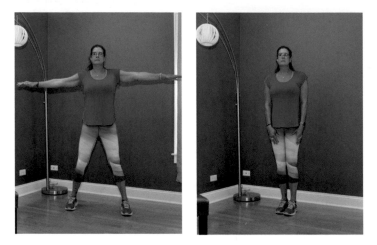

STEP OUTS

With the weight on the right leg take the left leg out to the side while bringing your arms up. Touch the toe to the floor and bring the leg back in, once again touching the toe. Repeat for 30 seconds on each side.

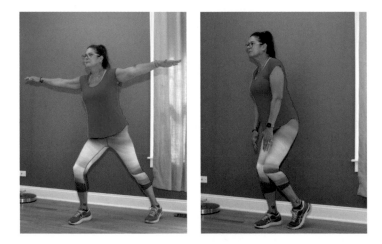

STEP TOUCH AND LIFT

Take a step to the right. Bring the left foot next to the right and press up on the calves as you take the arms overhead. Repeat, alternating sides for 30 seconds. You can also add a jump on the lift part of the exercise if you want more intensity.

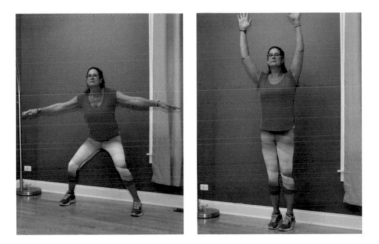

CROSSOVER KNEE LIFTS

Put your weight on the right leg and take your left leg out to the side with the arms up and at a diagonal. Bring the left knee up while pulling your arms down towards the left hip, squeezing your abs. Repeat for 30 seconds and switch sides.

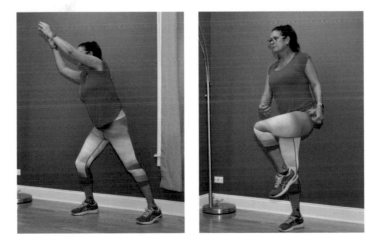

STRAIGHT LEG KICKS

Stand next to a chair or wall if needed for balance. Keep the weight on the left foot and lift the leg straight up in front of you. Keep a slight bend in the knee and only go as high as is comfortable for you and your flexibility. Repeat for 30 seconds on this side before switching sides. You should feel a gentle stretch.

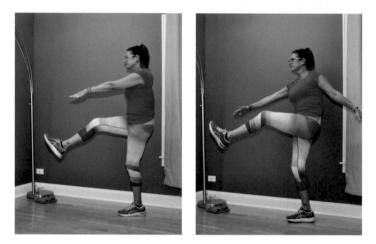

INNER THIGH HEEL LIFTS

Stand with feet about hip-width apart. Bend the left knee and bring the heel up and across your body, bringing the right arm towards the heel. If you need to balance, hold on to a chair or the wall and repeat on the same leg for 30 seconds before switching sides. For more intensity, alternate heel lifts for 30 seconds.

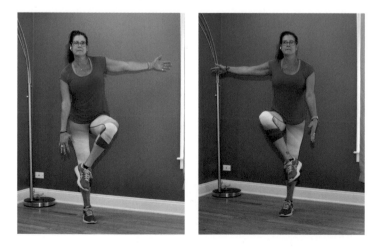

SQUAT WITH CROSSED ARM LIFT

Bend the knees and send the hips back into a squat while crossing the arms in front of your knees. Go as low as you can and push through the heels to stand, taking the arms up and overhead. Repeat for 30 seconds.

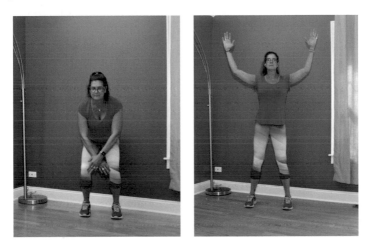

MARCH WITH CHEST SQUEEZE

Begin with the arms bent, the hands at ear level and perpendicular to the floor. Squeeze the arms together and out while marching in place. Repeat for 30 seconds.

Repeat the entire sequence of exercises, one after the other for 1 to 3 circuits, depending on how warmed up you feel.

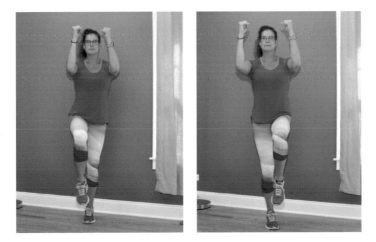

COOL DOWN

Like the warm-up and your actual workout, the cool down is essential for getting your body back to where it was before exercise. Taking a little time to slow your body down with simple movements can help you recover your pre-exercise heart rate and blood pressure.

This can be as simple as just walking around the house to catch your breath or doing the following exercises that allow you to cool down and stretch the muscles you've worked.

The Workout: Cool Down
Equipment: None
How it Works: Do each exercise one after the other, completing as many circuits as you like.

STEP TOUCH

Step out to the right side as far as you can, bringing the arms up and out to shoulder level. Bring the left foot next to the right, touch the floor, and then step back to the left, repeating the move while alternating sides for 30 seconds.

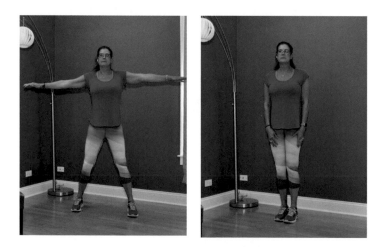

SIDE TO SIDE LUNGE

Stand with the feet wide and tip forward a bit, supporting your upper body with the hands on the thighs. Gently lunge to the right, feeling a stretch in the left inner thigh. Move back and forth between sides for 30 seconds.

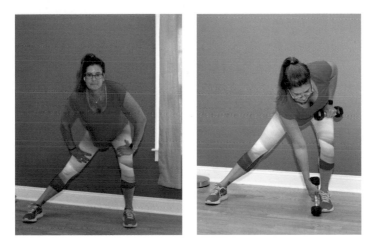

CALF STRETCH

Using a chair or wall for balance, bend the right knee and step the left foot back with a straight leg. Gently push the left heel towards the floor to stretch the calves. Hold for 30 seconds and repeat on the other side.

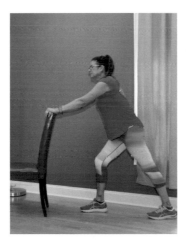

HAMSTRING STRETCH

Using a chair for balance, take the left foot forward, resting on the heel. Bend the back knee and gently press forward to stretch the back of the thigh. Hold for 30 seconds and repeat on the other side.

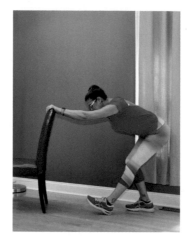

SEATED HIP STRETCH

Sit tall in a chair, abs engaged. Cross the left ankle over the right knee and gently press forward until you feel a stretch in the hips and outer thigh. Hold for 30 seconds and repeat on the other side.

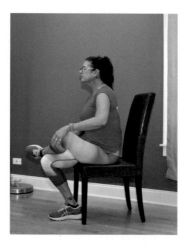

UPPER BACK STRETCH

Sit tall in a chair and lace your fingers together, stretching the arms straight. Pull the abs in, round the back, and stretch the arms out until you feel a stretch between your shoulder blades. Hold for 30 seconds.

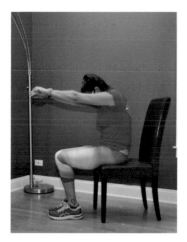

TOWEL CHEST STRETCH

Sit tall and hold a small rolled-up towel in both hands, palms wide. Take the arms up and gently pull on either side of the towel as you take the arms back to stretch the chest. Hold for 30 seconds.

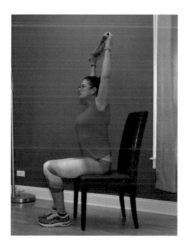

FLEXIBILITY WORKOUT

The Workout: Flexibility
Equipment: Resistance band
How it Works: Do each stretch for the suggested time, pulling gently for each muscle group

REAR LEG STRETCH

Lie down and loop the resistance band over the leg foot. Take it straight up in the air and very gently pull the handles so that you feel a stretch in the back of the legs. Hold for about 30 seconds and switch sides. This should feel relaxing.

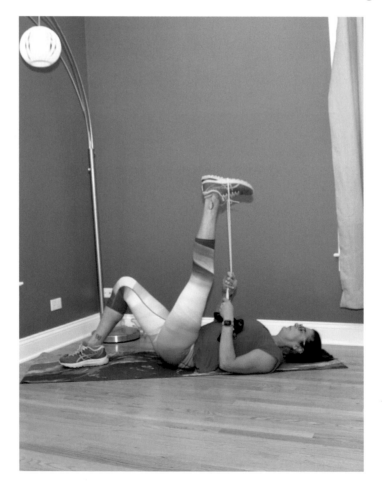

INNER THIGH STRETCH

Lying down, loop the band over the leg foot and gently take it out to the left side, supporting the leg with one hand. Only go as far as feels comfortable. Hold for about 30 seconds and then switch sides.

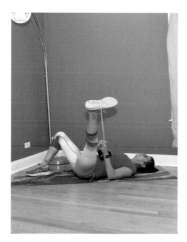

SPINE STRETCH

If you have any back issues, you might want to skip this one or ask your doctor about it. Lying on your back, bend the right knee and place your right foot on your left knee. Use your left hand to very gently rotate your body towards the left, stretching the spine. Try to keep your shoulders on the floor. Hold for about 30 seconds and repeat on the other side.

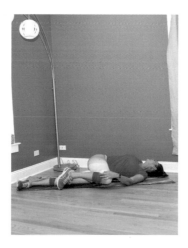

SHOULDER STRETCH

Seated or standing, take the right arm across the chest, drop the shoulder, and gently press the arm in with the left arm. Hold for about 30 seconds and switch sides.

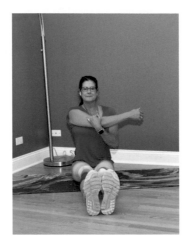

LAT STRETCH

This stretch is for the side of your back. Hold the resistance band in the right hand just behind the body as you sit with the feet crossed or the legs in front of you. Hold the band on the floor as you stretch the left arm up, stretching through the back. Hold for about 30 seconds before switching sides.

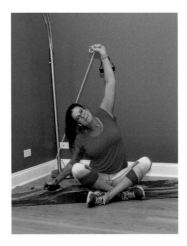

TRICEPS STRETCH

Seated or standing, take the right arm straight up and bend the elbow, bringing the right hand behind the head. Use the left arm to gently pull the elbow in to stretch the back of the arms. Hold for about 30 seconds and switch sides.

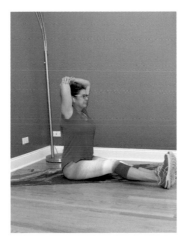

CHEST STRETCH

Sit on the floor or on a chair and hold a resistance band in both hands. Open the hands as you take the band up and slightly behind the head to stretch the chest. Hold for about 30 seconds and release.

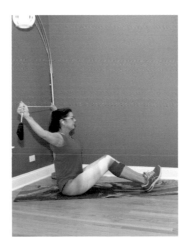

CAT COW STRETCH

On the hands and knees, inhale as you arch the back, taking the hips down and the chest forward. As you exhale, round the back up towards the ceiling, holding the abs in. Continue smoothly moving through each phase for 12 reps.

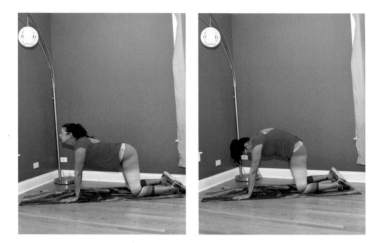

CORE WORKOUT

While you have some core exercises for each total body workout, this provides a focused workout for your core, which includes your entire torso—the abs, back, pelvic area.

This workout can be done about three times a week, with at least a day in between.

WOODCHOP

Hold a weight or medicine ball in both hands with the feet together. Take the weight up and at a diagonal to the right side. Step out to the left and sweep the weight diagonally and to the left, squeezing the abs. Step back and repeat for all reps before switching sides. Suggested weight: medium to heavy.

   1 x 12 reps

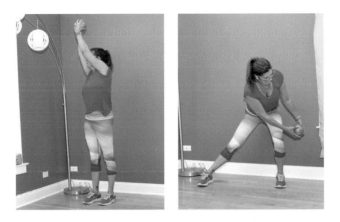

LUNGE WITH ROTATION

Hold a weight in both hands and step back with the right foot into a lunge. Make sure both knees bend and the back knee goes straight down to the floor. As you lunge, take the arms straight out and rotate the weight to the opposite side. Return to start and repeat on the other side. Suggested weight: medium to heavy.

   1 x 12 reps

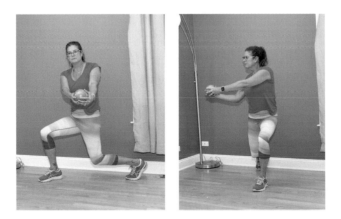

MEDICINE BALL SIDE CRUNCH

Hold a weight or a medicine ball in both hands with the arms straight up. Take the feet about shoulder-width apart and, keeping the abs braced, lean to the right as far as you can without moving the hips. Come back to center and repeat the move to the other side. Suggested weight: medium to heavy.

1 x 12 reps

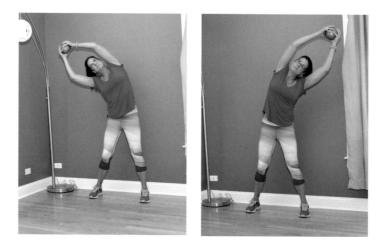

PLANK WITH KNEES

Get into a plank position, on the elbows and toes. You can also modify by staying on the knees or being on your hands and toes. Keep your back straight and your abs in and slowly lower your knees to the floor. Gently touch the knees and then press back up.

1 x 12 reps

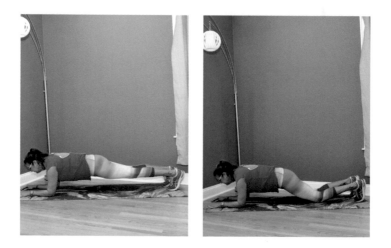

STRAIGHT LEG CRUNCH

Lie on your back on your mat and take one leg up in the air. Crunch the abs and lift the opposite hand to the foot as high as you can. Lower and repeat for all reps before switching sides. You can modify by keeping the knee bent.

1 x 12 reps

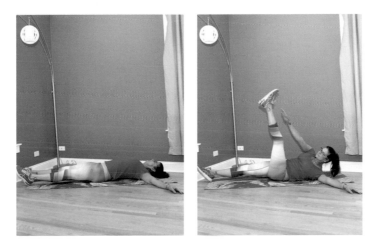

BRIDGE WITH A LEG DROP

Lying on your back on the floor, bend the knees and lift the hips so that you're in a bridge position. Keeping that position, straighten the left leg up. Gently and slowly take the left leg just a few inches towards the left side of the floor, feeling your core brace. Bring it back to center and repeat before switching sides. If this feels uncomfortable, do the basic bridge or avoid the leg drop and just take the leg up and down.

1 x 12 reps

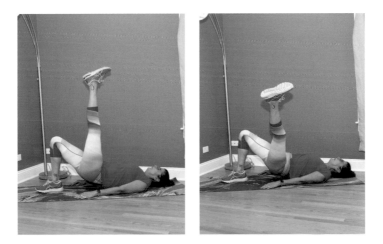

Chapter 8

Weeks 1 & 2—Let's Get Started

For your first couple of weeks we'll be getting used to exercise and figure out how much weight to choose for each exercise. Previously, I suggested you have about three sets of weights—light, medium, and heavy.

The amount of weight you use will change as you get stronger and it could change from week to week depending on how you're feeling and your energy.

SUGGESTED WORKOUT SCHEDULE:

Day 1: Total Body Strength Circuit 1/Cool down
Day 2: Cardio HIIT or LISS
Day 3: Rest and active movement
Day 4: Total Body Strength Circuit 2/Cool down
Day 5: Rest and flexibility
Day 6: Core workout and flexibility
Day 7: Cardio of your choice

The Workout: Total Body Strength Circuit 1
Equipment: Light to medium dumbbells, a chair, and a mat
How it Works: Do each exercise one after the other, completing 1 to 2 circuits. If you do more than one circuit, rest for about 30 seconds to a minute in between circuits. If you need to.

LUNGE WITH LATERAL RAISE

For balance, stand next to a wall or hold on to a chair if needed. Hold a weight in the left hand and step the left foot back about three feet in a staggered stance. Bend the knees and lower into a lunge, taking the back knee straight down to the floor. At the same time, lift the right arm with the weight straight up to the side as you lunge. Press back up and repeat before switching sides. Suggested weight: light.

   1 x 12 reps

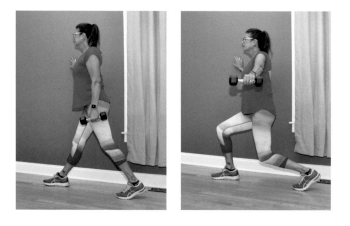

SIT AND STAND WITH TOWEL SQUEEZE

Put a chair behind you (sit down first to test it!) and hold a rolled-up towel straight up in front of you, standing in front of the chair. Squeeze the towel open to engage the back. Holding the towel like that, lower into a squat and briefly sit on the chair. Stand and repeat.

   1 x 12 reps

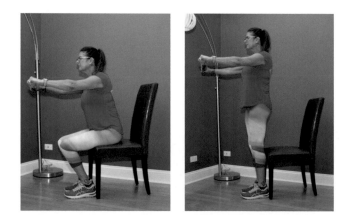

TOWEL SIDES

Hold on to a chair for balance if needed and place a small folded towel under the right foot. Holding on to the chair, slide the left foot back while bending the front knee in a lunge. Slide the foot back in and repeat.

   1 x 12 reps

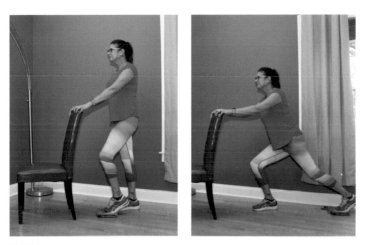

SQUAT AND CURL

Holding weights in both hands, step out to the right into a squat as you curl the weights up in a bicep curl. Lower the weights, step together, and (optional) do another biceps curl. Continue squatting to either side and curling the arms up. For more stability, take out the steps and just do a regular squat. You can also do a squat first, then stand and do a biceps curl for a modification. Suggested weight: medium to heavy.

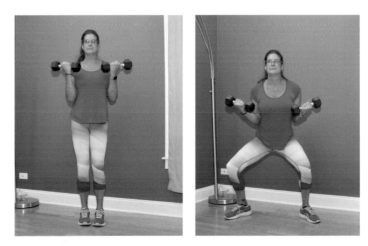

REAR LUNGE WITH ROW

Hold weights in both hands with the feet together. Step the right leg back into a straight-leg lunge, while pulling the elbows up to the torso, squeezing the back muscles. Step back and take the left leg back into a straight-leg lunge and pull the elbows up to the torso in a rowing motion. Continue alternating sides. For a modification, do the step back first, then step together and do the row separately. You can also do it without the weights. Suggested weight: medium to heavy.

1 x 12 reps

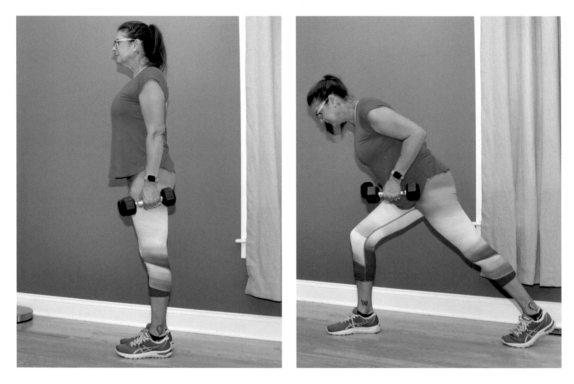

SQUAT WITH ONE ARM PRESS

Start with the feet hip-distance apart, holding weights in both hands, just over the shoulders. Lower into a squat, sending the hips back and keeping the abs engaged. Press through the heel to stand up and press the right arm up in a shoulder press. Repeat, alternating arms. For a modification, hold the weights at your sides and do a squat. Stand and take one arm up overhead. Suggested weight: light to medium.

  1 x 12 reps

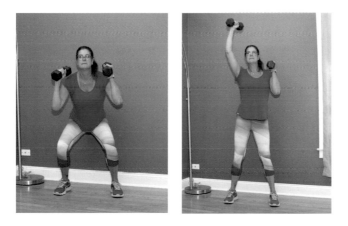

TRICEPS EXTENSIONS WITH HEEL TOUCH

Begin with the feet together, holding a weight in both hands with the elbows bent, the weight behind your head. Extend the arms as you take the right heel forward. Return to start, lowering the arms behind the head and stepping the heel back. Continue, alternating sides. For a modification, take out the heel taps, or do the heel tap first, step back, and then do the triceps extension. Suggested weight: medium to heavy.

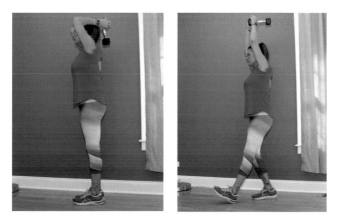

GOOD MORNINGS

Stand with feet together and hands cupping the head, elbows out. You can also hold a light weight behind the head for more intensity. Tip from the hips with knees slightly bent and lower the torso until it's parallel to the floor, back flat, and shoulders back. Squeeze the back to lift back up.

   1 x 12 reps

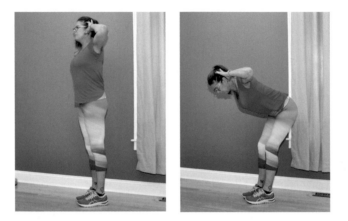

STANDING CROSSOVER CRUNCHES

Begin with the feet wide facing the right wall, hands on the head and elbows back. Bring the left knee in as you cross the right elbow towards the knee. Lower and repeat before switching sides.

   1 x 12 reps

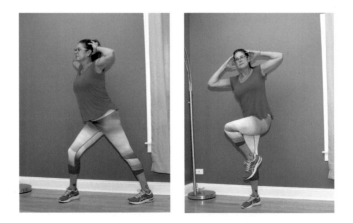

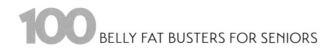

PUSHUPS

Get on all fours on the floor and walk the hands out until you have a straight line from the head to your heels. Bend the elbows and lower into a pushup as low as you can go, then press back up. You can choose this version or the modified version on the hands and knees, shown here. You can also do a wall pushup where you stand about three feet from the wall with hands shoulder-width apart.

 1 x 12 reps

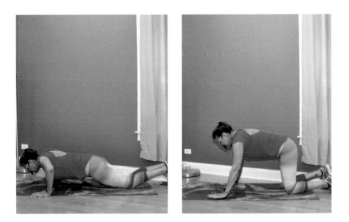

BIRD DOG

Get on your hands and knees, hands directly under the shoulders and the knees directly under the hips. Lift the right arm straight out at the same time you lift the left leg up . . . in other words, opposite arm and leg. If your balance is off, just lift one limb at a time. Lower and repeat on the other side.

 1 x 12 reps

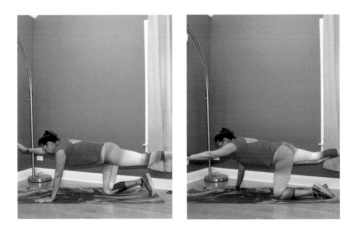

CRUNCH WITH HEEL PUSH

Lie on the floor on your back, knees bent, and hands behind the head. Flex the heels and crunch the upper body up as you push into the floor with your heels. Lower and repeat. Try not to pull on your neck. This can be a very small move.

1 x 12 reps

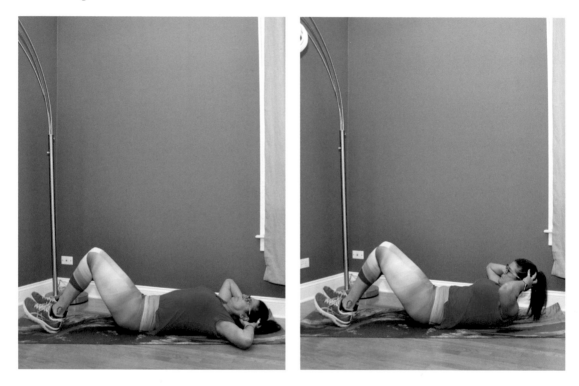

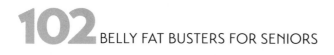

Chapter 9
Weeks 3 & 4—Getting Stronger

You've built a strong foundation during the first two weeks, and now we're building on that foundation with new and different complex exercises.

These exercises have a lot of moving parts, so take your time and practice each part of the movement before you pick up the weights. Good form should be your first priority and many of these exercises involve multiple muscle groups and joints.

Give yourself time to learn the movements and then add weights when you're ready.

SUGGESTED WORKOUT SCHEDULE:

Day 1: Total Body Strength Circuit 2/Cool down
Day 2: Cardio HIIT or LISS
Day 3: Rest and active movement
Day 4: Total Body Strength Circuit 2/Cool down
Day 5: Rest and active movement
Day 6: Core workout and flexibility
Day 7: Cardio of your choice, flexibility

The Workout: Total Body Strength Circuit 2
Equipment: Light to medium dumbbells, a chair, and a mat
How it Works: Do each exercise one after the other, completing 1 to 2 circuits. If you do more than one circuit, rest for about 30 seconds to a minute in between circuits if you need to.

SQUAT WITH OVERHEAD PRESS

Step out to the side, holding weights just over the shoulders with the elbows bent. Step back to starting position and press the weights overhead. Repeat the move to the other side and continue alternating side squats with overhead presses. For a modification, don't do the step out, just do a regular squat. You can also squat, stand, and then do the overhead press instead of doing them together. Suggested weight: medium.

1 x 12 reps

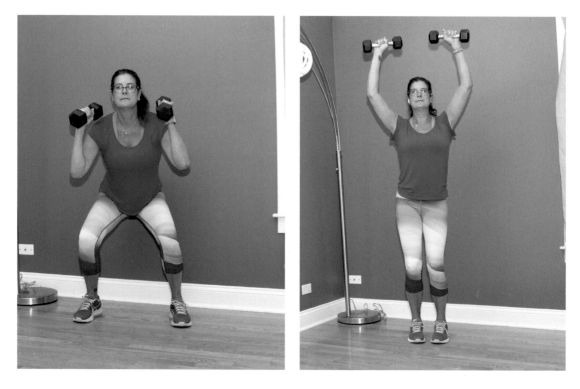

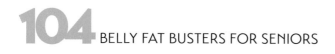

LUNGE WITH TRICEPS EXTENSIONS

Stand in a staggered stance, with the right foot forward and the left foot back in a static lunge. Hold a weight in the right hand, straight up over the shoulder. Hold on to a chair or wall for balance. Staying in the lunge position, bend the elbow and lower the weight behind the head. Press the arm back up, staying in the lunge, and repeat for all reps before switching sides. For a modification, take the lunge out and stand with the feet together. Suggested weight: light to medium.

1 x 12 reps

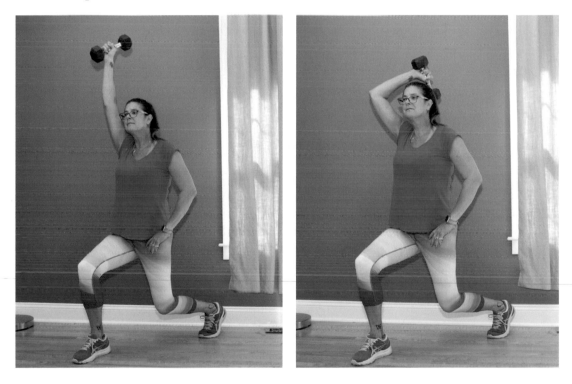

DEADLIFT TO DUMBBELL ROW

Stand with feet hip-distance apart, holding weights in front of the thighs. Tip from the hips with a flat back and abs in and lower the weights towards the shins. Keep the weights close to the legs like you're shaving them. Only go as far as your flexibility allows. At the bottom of the movement, turn the hands so they're facing in and pull the elbows up into a row, squeezing both sides of the back. Lower the weights, squeeze the glutes to stand up, and repeat. If this bothers your back, you can sit on a chair and do a double arm row without the deadlift. Suggested weight: medium to heavy.

1 x 12 reps

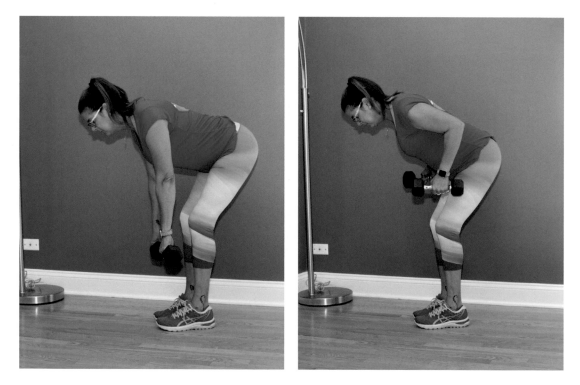

DUMBBELL SWING WITH SHOULDER PRESS

Hold weights in both hands and lower into a squat. Swing the weights between the knees and press up, taking the weights overhead. Lower the weights to shoulder level in a shoulder press. Press the weights back up and then swing them down again. Suggest weight: light to medium.

1 x 12 reps

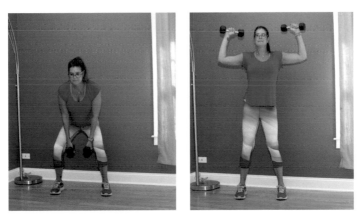

WIDE SQUAT CHEST SQUEEZE

Hold a weight or medicine ball in both hands with the feet wide, toes angled out. Squeeze the weight as you bend the knees into a wide squat, pushing the weight straight out in front of you. Stand straight up and bring the weight in towards the chest. Repeat trying to keep the same amount of pressure on the weight. For a modification, do the chest squeeze out and in separately from the squat. You can also do a regular squat if the wide squats don't work for you. Suggested weight: light to medium.

1 x 12 reps

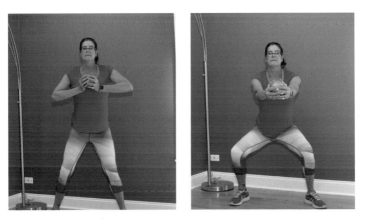

PUSHUPS

On the hands and knees (easier) or toes (harder), walk the hands out until your back is flat, hands a little wider than shoulders. Bend the elbows, keep the abs engaged, and lower into a pushup. Press back up and repeat. Remember you can do wall pushups if you need a modification.

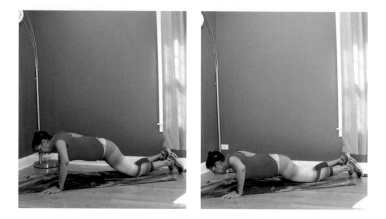

CHEST FLY WITH HEEL DROPS

Lie on the floor and hold weights in both hands overhead, palms facing each other. Bring the knees up (optional) until they're at 90-degree angles—keep the feet on the floor if this feels uncomfortable. Otherwise, open the arms and take the weights out towards the floor, elbows slightly bent. At the same time, take one foot to the floor. Bring the arms back and the foot in and repeat, alternating sides. For modifications, leave the legs straight up, bend them, or keep them on the floor. Suggested weight: light to medium.

1 x 12 reps

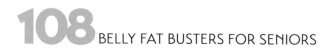

BAND WOODCHOP

Stand with the feet wide and loop the resistance band under one foot, holding on to both handles with the hands at a diagonal, next to the left thigh. Rotate the body in the other direction, taking the arms up and to the right. Repeat for all reps before switching sides. For a modification, you can stand on one end of the band and just hold one handle at a time.

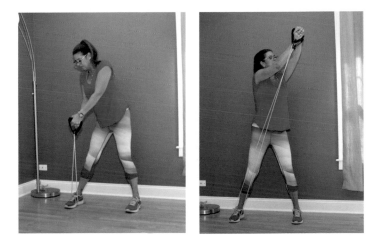

BACK EXTENSIONS

Lie on your stomach on the floor and place the hands on the floor in front of you with the elbows bent. Press up, lifting the chest off the floor, using the hands just for support. For added intensity, lift the legs off the floor at the same time. Lower and repeat.

1 x 12 reps

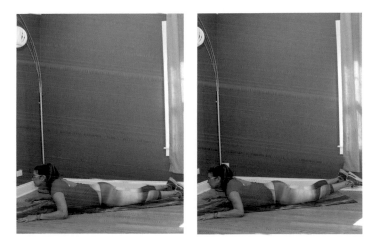

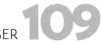

Chapter 10
Weeks 5 & 6—Building Muscle

Now we ramp things up again with some new exercises, still focusing on compound exercises and building strength, balance, and flexibility.

These moves are more dynamic, involving your entire body. They may feel challenging, so feel free to take more time at previous levels if these moves feel too difficult. I've added in modifications just like in previous workouts so, at this point, you probably have a good idea of how to change things so that you feel stable and safe.

You can also keep doing previous workouts or swap out exercises if something doesn't work for you. At this point, you'll know more about your body and how much you can push it without injury or pain. Just keep moving. Everything counts!

SUGGESTED WORKOUT SCHEDULE:

Day 1: Total Body Strength Circuit 3/Cool down
Day 2: Cardio HIIT or LISS
Day 3: Rest and active movement
Day 4: Total Body Strength Circuit 3/Cool down
Day 5: Core and flexibility
Day 6: Cardio HIIT or LISS
Day 7: Rest and active movement

The Workout: Total Body Strength Circuit 3
Equipment: Light to medium dumbbells, a resistance band, a mat
How it Works: Do each exercise one after the other, completing 1 to 3 circuits. If you do more than one circuit and you need to rest for about 30 seconds to a minute in between circuits, you should do so.

REVERSE LUNGE WITH STRAIGHT ARM OVERHEAD

Begin with the feet together and hold a weight in the left hand. Take that weight straight up over the shoulder. Hold on to a wall or chair for balance if needed. Keeping the arm straight up, step back into a lunge with the left leg. Make sure you take the knees straight down rather than forward. Step back and repeat all reps on the right side before switching sides. For modifications, do a regular lunge. You can also step back with the arm down, step forward with the feet together, and then take the arm up. Suggested weight: light to heavy.

1 x 12 reps

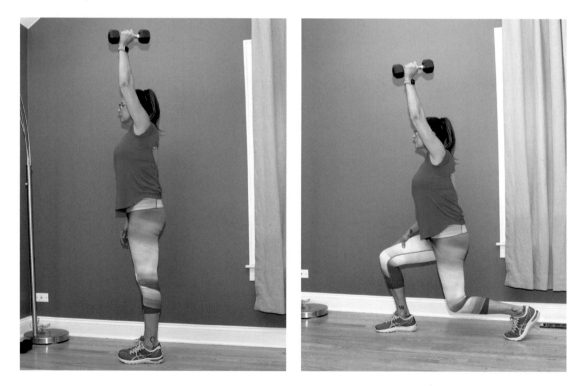

SQUAT AND SNATCH

Stand with feet about shoulder-width apart with a weight on the floor between your feet. Lower into a squat, sending your hips back, and grab the weight. Press into the heels to push up in a dynamic movement, using your lower body to gain momentum as you lift the weight, keeping it close to your body. As the dumbbell reaches your shoulder, flip your elbow so that the weight is facing out and lift it straight up. Try to focus on using the lower body to push the weight up rather than just your arm. Do all reps on one side before switching sides. This is a complex move, so to modify, you can put the weight on a chair and do each move separately: Squat to pick up the weight. Pull the weight up in front of the chest. Flip the elbow so that the weight faces out and press up. You can also completely skip this exercise if you feel uncomfortable. Suggested weight: light.

1 x 12 reps

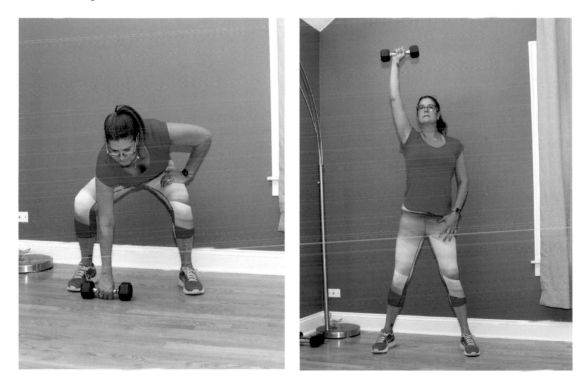

SQUAT WITH BAND ROW

Loop your resistance band under both feet and, if you need more tension, wrap the band around your hands. Bend the knees and send the hips back into a squat, keeping tension on the bend. At the bottom of the movement pull the elbows up, squeezing either side of the back. Lower the arms and stand up. For a modification, just stand on one side of the resistance band and hold the other handle in your hand. You can place the other hand on your thigh for support as you squat, then row, then stand.

   1 x 12 reps

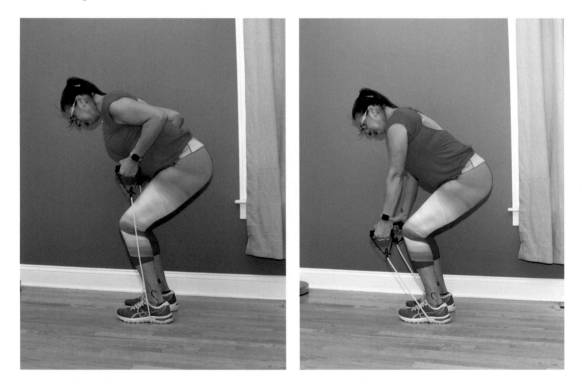

STATIC LUNGE WITH BAND SHOULDERS

Loop the resistance band under the left foot and wrap the band around your hands if you need more tension. Step the right foot back and bend both knees into a lunge, making sure the back knee goes straight towards the floor as low as you can. Hold that position and then lift the arms straight up in front of you and then out to the side. Repeat all reps before switching sides. For a modification, do the move without the lunge and/or do the exercise one arm at a time while holding on to a chair or wall for balance.

  1 x 12 reps

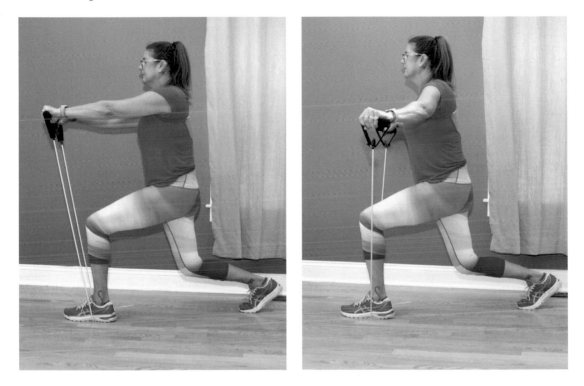

BAND STEP OUT BICEPS

Loop the resistance band under both feet and wrap the band around your hands for more resistance. Step out to the right into a squat and curl the arms up to your shoulders, squeezing the biceps. Step back in a repeat for all reps before switching sides. For a modification, just do a regular squat with a biceps curl. You can also do the curls one arm at a time instead of together.

1 x 12 reps

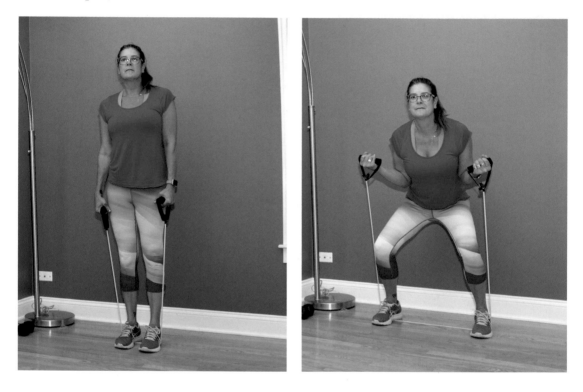

BAND ONE LEG TRICEPS EXTENSIONS

Fold your resistance band in half and hold the top with the right hand and grab on below that with the left hand. You might need to test the tension of the band to find what works best for you. Lift one foot off the ground or rest on your heel and hold that position as you straighten the right hand, squeezing the back of the arm. Return to start and repeat for all reps before switching sides. For a modification, do the triceps extension and then the leg lift, or take out the leg portion of the movement.

1 x 12 reps

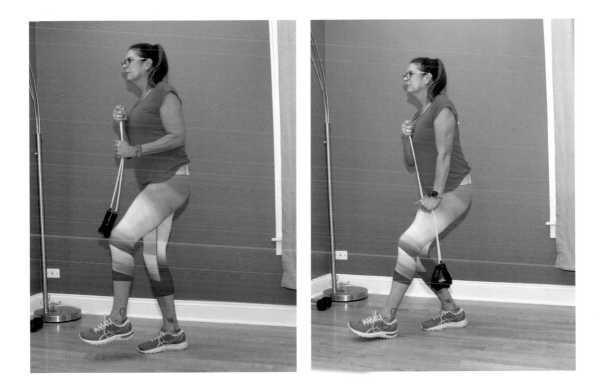

CLOSE GRIP BENCH PRESS

Lie on your back on the floor or on a bench if you have one and hold weights in both hands, palms facing in and with elbows bent and right next to your torso. Press the weights straight up over the chest, feeling the movement in your chest, shoulders, and triceps. Lower the weight down, just barely touching the floor, and repeat. The idea is that your elbows stay close to the body and you press the weight straight up with the palms facing in. Suggested weight: light to medium.

    1 x 12 reps

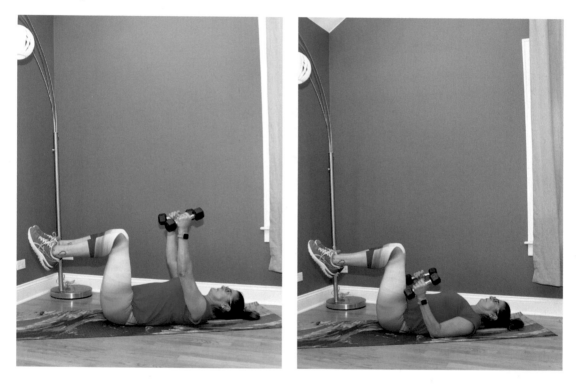

PUSHUP WITH LEG LIFT

Start in a pushup position, with the hands a bit wider than your shoulders. You can be on your knees or toes. Lift one leg off the floor keeping the knee bent. Lower into a pushup, keeping the leg up. Continue doing pushups, alternating leg lifts. As a modification, do regular pushups without the leg movement or wall pushups.

1 x 12 reps

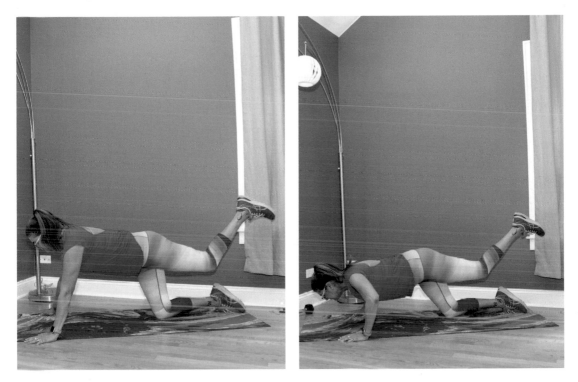

CHEST FLY WITH LEG DROPS

Begin on the floor holding weights in both hands, palms facing in straight up over the chest. Take the legs up in the air (optional). Open the arms out to the sides, elbows slightly bent in a chest fly. At the same time, take one leg towards the floor. Bring the arms and leg back to start and repeat, alternating legs. Make sure your abs are engaged to protect your lower back. For modifications, keep the legs straight up, bend the knees, or keep the legs on the floor with the knees bent.

   1 x 12 reps

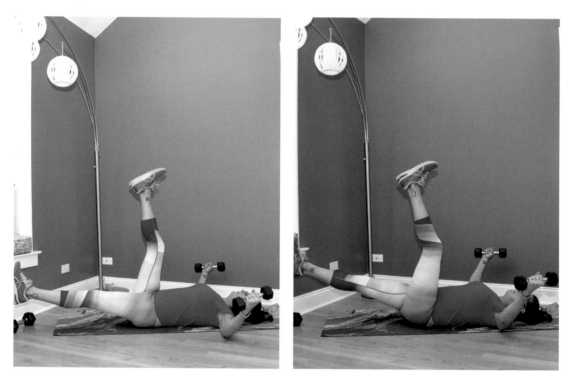

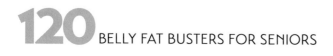

PLANK WITH KNEE LIFTS

Get into a plank position on the elbows and toes or on the knees if you need a modification. You can also do this move on your hands, which is a little easier. Try to keep the hips down so that your body is in a straight line. If you're on the knees, hold the plank for 30 to 60 seconds. If you're on your toes, drop the knees down and up. For another modification, you can take the hips up a little more towards the ceiling and work your way up to a flat position.

  1 x 12 reps

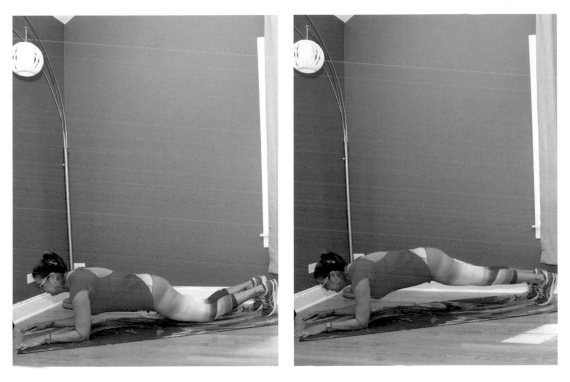

RUSSIAN TWIST

Get into a seated position on the floor with the knees bent and the spine straight. Hold a weight or a medicine ball in both hands, brace the abs, and lean back a few inches. Rotate the torso to the left, bringing the weight towards the floor. Return to your starting position and rotate to the other side. Continue alternating sides. For a modification, you can sit up straight or you can do this seated in a chair, rotating from side to side. Suggested weight: light to medium.

   1 x 12 reps

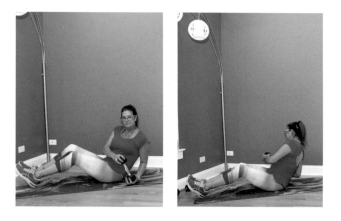

BRIDGE

Lie on your back on the floor with the knees bent and arms by your sides. Squeeze the glutes to lift the hips up so that your body is in a straight line. Lower and repeat. For more intensity, you can hold weights on the hips.

   1 x 16 reps

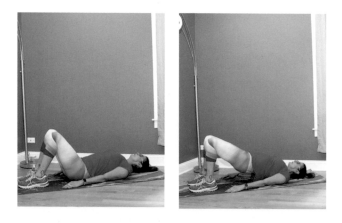

Chapter 11
Weeks 7 & 8—Making Changes

If you've made it this far, you're doing amazing. Remember that this is your workout program, so make it work for you.

We're progressing further for the next couple of weeks and introducing an exercise ball to the mix along with some brand-new exercises to challenge you and keep things interesting. The exercise ball adds an element of instability, which is perfect for working on balance. But, it can have a learning curve, so always make sure you feel safe. Keep something nearby you can hold on to as needed and remember, you can do the exercises without the ball or go back to previous workouts or take extra rest days as needed.

Remember, there are modifications for every exercise and you can also skip anything you don't like.

Every week won't be perfect and there are times when life intervenes. Don't feel discouraged if that happens. Just lace on your shoes and do some kind of movement. Deal?

SUGGESTED WORKOUT SCHEDULE:

Day 1: Total Body Strength Circuit 4/Cool down
Day 2: Rest and active movement
Day 3: Cardio HIIT or LISS
Day 4: Total Body Strength Circuit 4/Cool down
Day 5: Core and flexibility
Day 6: Cardio HIIT or LISS
Day 7: Rest and active movement

The Workout: Total Body Strength Circuit 4

Equipment: Light to medium dumbbells, an exercise ball, a resistance band, a mat

How it Works: Do each exercise one after the other, completing 1 to 3 circuits. If you do more than one circuit, rest for about 30 seconds to a minute in between circuits.

BALL SQUAT

Place the ball against the wall and, if you can do so safely, grab a pair of dumbbells. This can be challenging so you might want to keep a chair nearby with your weights so you can pick them up safely. Holding the weights, lean against the ball with your upper body, and slowly walk your feet out just a bit until you're leaning against the ball. Lower into a squat and push into the heels to stand up. This will challenge your balance and core. As a modification, leave the weights out. You can also do regular squats without the ball, since that can be hard to use at first. Suggested weight: none or light to medium.

1 x 12 reps

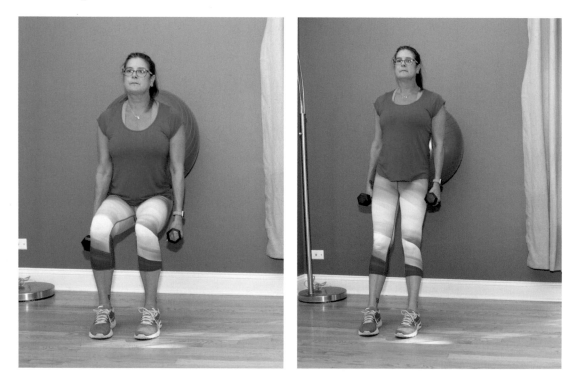

CURTSY LUNGE WITH A SWING

Hold a weight in the right hand with feet together. Cross the right leg behind the left side of your body as if you're doing a curtsy. Step back in and swing the weight up to shoulder level. Repeat all reps before switching sides. As a modification, hold on to a chair for balance and you can also just do the squat without swinging the weight. Suggested weight: light to medium.

1 x 12 reps

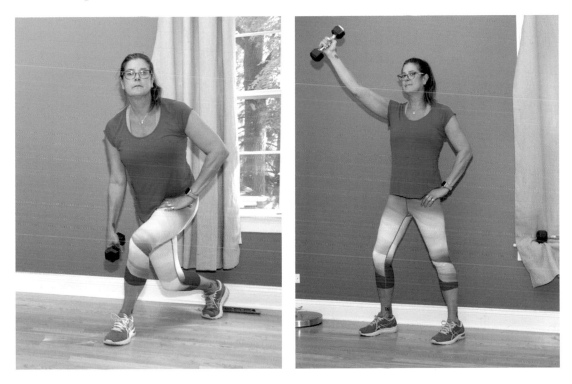

SIDE TO SIDE LUNGE

Start with the feet wide and toes at a slight angle, holding weights in both hands. Bend the right knee while keeping the left knee straight into a side lunge while bringing the weight in the left hand towards the floor as low as you can, but not so much that you tweak your back. Return to start and repeat on the other side. Continue alternating sides for all reps. As a modification, you can hold one weight in the right hand and do a side lunge to the right, keeping all reps on the same side before switching. Suggested weight: light to medium.

1 x 12 reps

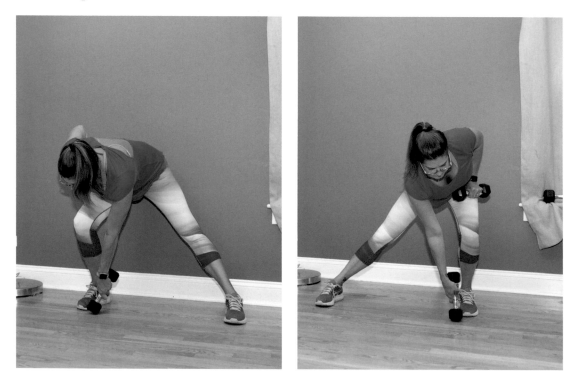

SIDE LUNGE TO ROW

With the feet wide, hold a weight in the left hand and bend the right knee into a side lunge, left leg straight. You may need a chair or wall for balance for the next part of this exercise. Lift the left leg up in a side leg lift while pulling the elbow up to the torso into a row. Lower the leg and the arm and repeat for all reps before switching sides. As a modification, take the leg lift out, or do the leg lift first, lower, and then do the row. Suggested weight: medium to heavy.

   1 x 12 reps

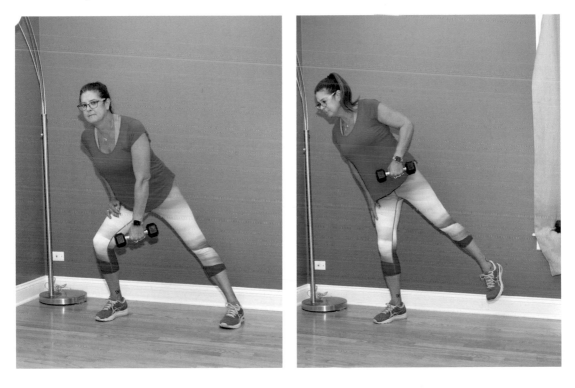

SQUAT WITH A ROTATING PRESS

Hold one weight in both hands, feet wide. Lower into a squat, sending the hips towards the back wall. As you push back up, rotate to the right, pivoting on the feet and taking the weight up overhead. Return to the starting position and alternate sides for all reps. As a modification, you can do the whole exercise without a weight, or take out the rotation and do a regular squat. Suggested weight: medium to heavy.

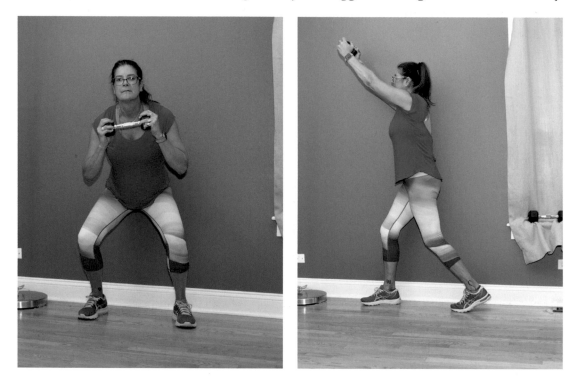

STEP BACK WITH REVERSE FLY

Hold weights in both hands with the feet together. Step back with the left leg, tip from the hips with a flat back and abs in to about a 45-degree angle. Lift the weight up to the side, squeezing the shoulder blades and feeling it in the upper back. Step the foot back in and repeat on the other side, this time lifting the other arm up. Continue alternating sides for all reps. As a modification, you can do all reps on the same side before switching, or you can keep the feet together and just do the reverse fly. You can also do this seated if this bothers your back. Suggested weight: light to medium.

1 x 12 reps

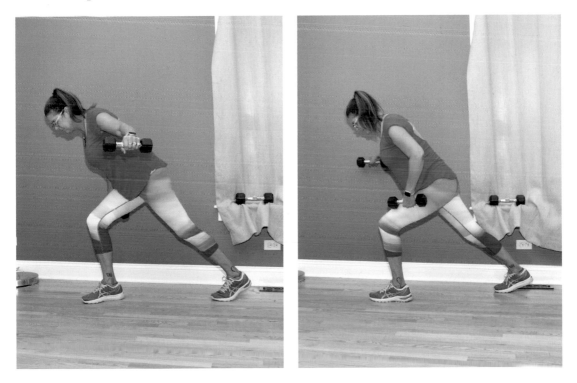

DEADLIFTS WITH BICEPS CURLS

This one is complex, so you'll get some modifications. Loop a resistance band under the left foot and take that foot forward so you're in a staggered stance, knees slightly bent. Wrap the band around your hands if you need more tension. Tip from the hips, back flat and abs in, lowering into a one-legged deadlift. Stand up, pushing into the heel and now step back into a lunge with the right foot while doing a biceps curl. Return to start and repeat all reps on one side before switching sides. As a modification, you can separate the exercises, doing the deadlifts all at once and then the lunges with biceps curls all at once. You can also do all three separately if that's more comfortable.

1 x 12 reps

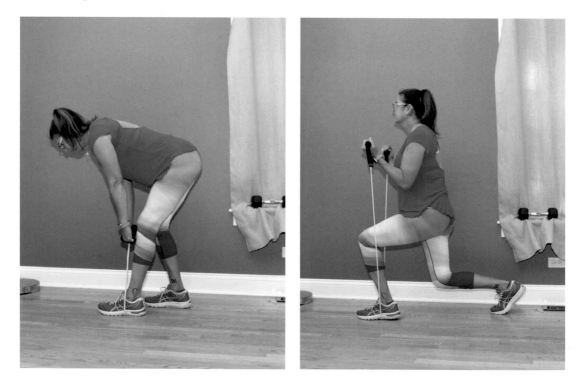

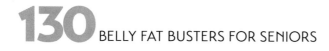

SHOULDER CRUNCH

Hold weights in both hands with the feet about shoulder-width apart. Take the right arm up at a 90-degree angle, weight at ear level. Lift the left knee as you bring the weight towards the knee, squeezing the abs. Lower and repeat on the other side. Continue alternating sides for all reps. As a modification, stay on one side of the body and hold on to a chair or wall for balance and then switch sides. You can also do the arm movement first and then lift the knee separately. Suggested weight: light.

1 x 12 reps

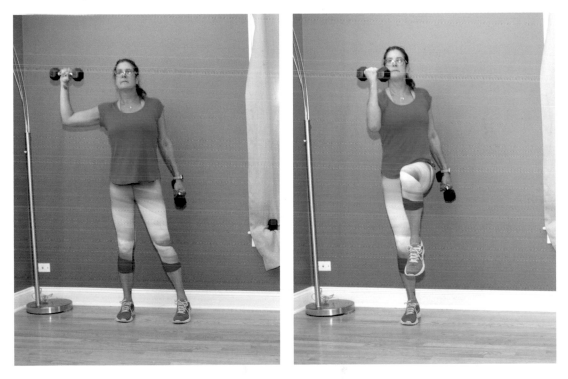

PUSHUP WITH LEG LIFT

Get into a pushup position, on the knees or toes. As you lower into a pushup, lift the left knee up. Push back up and repeat, alternating legs as you do pushups. You can also keep the knees down if this feels uncomfortable. As a modification, do regular pushups or wall pushups.

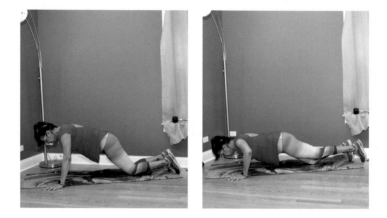

CHEST PRESS WITH LEGS

Lie on your back, on a mat or a bench with the legs straight up, holding weights in both hands. Press the weights straight up over the chest and, at the same time, bend the knees so they're at 90-degree angles (optional). Take the legs back up as you lower the weight and repeat for all reps. As a modification, keep the legs down, knees bent, and do regular chest presses. Suggest weight: medium to heavy.

1 x 12 reps

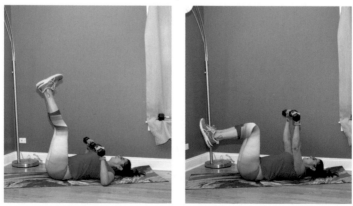

PLANK

Get into a plank position on the elbows and toes. If this isn't comfortable, you can get on your hands and knees. Whichever position you choose, hold it for as long as you can. You can rest the knees on the floor for short breaks as needed. Work on increasing the amount of time at each workout. As a modification, you can take your hips up slightly to take some of the pressure off, but work up to staying flat.

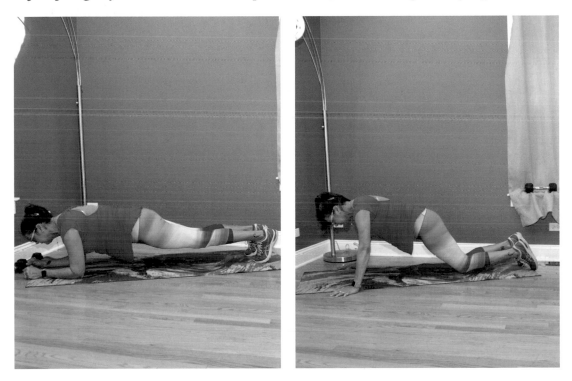

SIDE HIP LIFT

Lie down on your right side on a mat, resting on your elbow. Keep the knees bent and the hips stacked. You can rest the left hand on the floor if you need more support. Lift the hips up while keeping the knees on the floor, using the left hand for support or keeping it off the floor for more intensity. Repeat for all reps before switching sides. As a modification, use the left hand to push into the floor to help you lift up and keep the movement very small. Remember to keep the knees on the floor.

1 x 12 reps

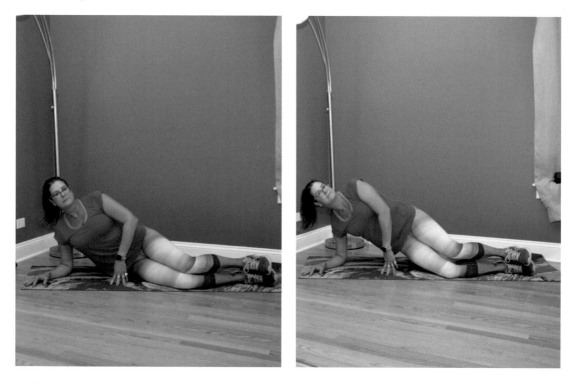

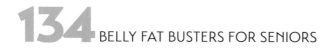

Chapter 12
Weeks 9 & 10—Getting There

You've made it this far, so now isn't the time to give up. This week we're doing even more work with the exercise ball. This is one of my favorite tools for building balance and core strength.

If you're not familiar with the ball, take your time and feel free to do the exercises without the ball if you need to. It takes some time to get used to, so you might want to be next to a wall or some other sturdy support for balance.

I've also switched he schedule to include an extra day of your Total Body Circuit Workout 5. It's completely up to you if you want to add that to your routine. Listen to your body and take time to focus on how you feel before adding more workouts.

SUGGESTED WORKOUT SCHEDULE:
Day 1: Total Body Strength Circuit 5/Cool down
Day 2: Rest and active movement
Day 3: Cardio HIIT or LISS
Day 4: Total Body Strength Circuit 5/Cool down
Day 5: Rest and flexibility
Day 6: Cardio HIIT or LISS and core
Day 7: Total Body Strength Circuit 5/Cool down

The Workout: Total Body Strength Circuit 5
Equipment: Light to medium dumbbells, an exercise ball, a resistance band, a mat
How it Works: Do each exercise one after the other, completing 1 to 3 circuits. If you do more than one circuit, you can rest for about 30 seconds to a minute in between circuits.

BALL SQUAT WITH FRONT RAISE

We're using the ball again for squats, so you might want to get a chair and put your weight on it next to you so you can safely pick it up. Place the ball against the wall and hold your weight in both hands, walking the feet out a bit so you're leaning against the ball. Bend the knees and lower into a squat, taking the knees to 90-degree angle or however low you can go. Press through the heels to stand up and take the weight straight up to shoulder level. Repeat for all reps. As a modification, don't use a weight or do the squat without the ball. Suggested weight: medium to heavy.

1 x 12 reps

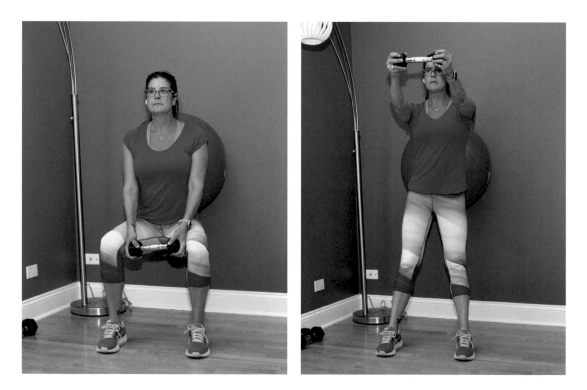

LUNGE WITH AN OVERHEAD PRESS

Hold weights in both hands at shoulder level and step back into a lunge with the right foot. As you lunge, press the weights overhead. Return to the starting position, lowering the weights, and repeat, alternating sides. As a modification, do the lunge first, then step back and press the weights overhead. You can also hold one weight in the right hand, hold on to a chair, and do all the lunges on that side before switching sides. Suggested weight: light to medium.

1 x 12 reps

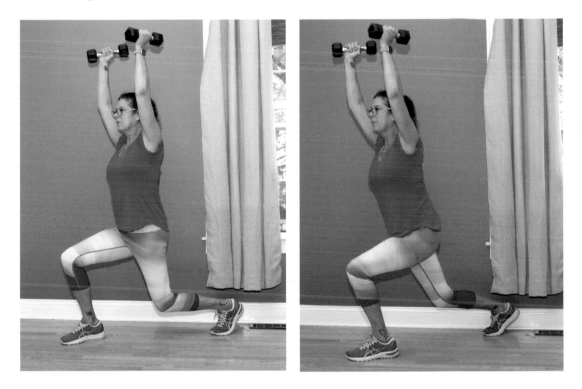

WIDE SQUAT BICEPS CURLS

Stand in a wide stance with the toes out at a slight angle. Hold weights in both hands. Lower into a wide squat as you curl the weights up in a biceps curl. Make sure your knees stay in line with your toes. Press into the heels to stand up and lower the weights. Repeat for all reps. As a modification, do the squat first, stand up, and then do the biceps curl. You can also do a regular squat if the wide squat doesn't work for you. Suggested weight: medium to heavy.

1 x 12 reps

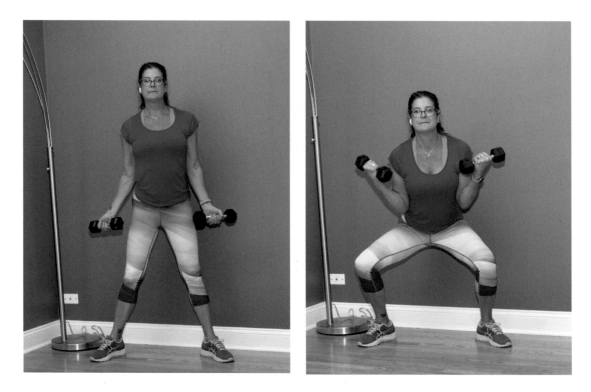

DUMBBELL ROW WITH A LEG LIFT

Hold a weight in the left hand and take the left leg back into a straight leg lunge. Pull the elbow up towards the torso, feeling it in your back as you lift the left leg up. Lower and repeat on the same side before switching. As a modification, take the leg lift out or hold on to a chair for balance and stability. Suggested weight: medium to heavy.

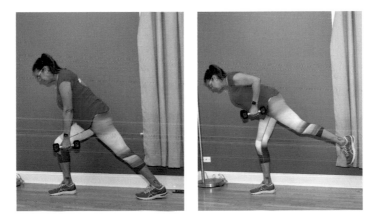

BAND SQUAT WITH ROTATING PRESS

Loop a resistance band under the right foot and hold handles in each hand. You may need to adjust where the band is to figure out the right amount of tension you need. Lower into a squat, holding the right hand at shoulder level. As you push up, rotate to the other side while pressing the band straight overhead. Repeat for all reps before switching sides. Note: You'll want to use your lightest band here. As a modification, just stand and press the band up without the rotation.

1 x 12 reps

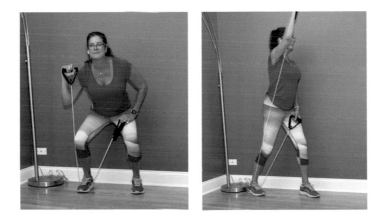

STEP BACK WITH REVERSE FLY

Hold a weight in one hand with the feet together. Step back with the left leg, and tip from the hips with a flat back and abs in to about a 45-degree angle. Lift the weight up to the side, squeezing the shoulder blades and feeling it in the upper back. Step the foot back in and repeat on the other side, this time lifting the other arm up. Continue alternating sides for all reps. As a modification, you can do all reps on the same side before switching, or you can keep the feet together and just do the reverse fly. You can also do this seated if this bothers your back. Suggested weight: light to medium.

1 x 12 reps

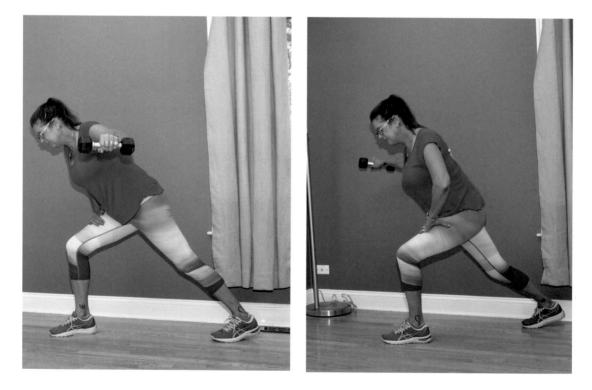

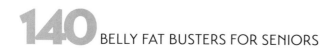

BALL CHEST PRESS

If this is the first time using your ball as a type of weight bench, keep a support nearby or do this exercise on the floor if you feel unbalanced. You can also practice this move without any weights just to get used to it. If you're using a ball, put your weights on the mat in front of you, sit on the ball, and slowly walk your body forward until your head and neck are supported on the ball. If you can safely do so, pick up your weights and start with elbows bent before pressing the weights straight up over the chest. Lower and repeat for all reps. Suggested weight: light to medium.

1 x 12 reps

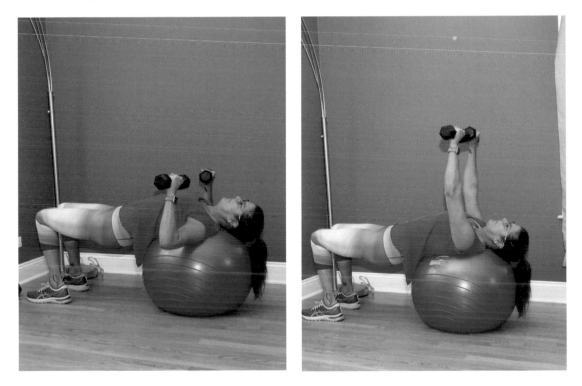

BALL ONE-ARMED FLY

This is another exercise that requires some balance, so use your best judgment as to whether you want to do this on the ball or on the floor. If you're new to the ball, keep a support nearby to help with balance. Begin holding one weight sitting on the ball. Keep the weight close to your chest and slowly walk your feet out until your upper back and neck are supported. Using a wall to help you walk forward on the ball helps. Take the weight in your left hand, straight up and, abs braced, lower the weight out to the side to torso level. Lift the weight back up and repeat for all reps before switching sides. Take your time, as this will really challenge your balance. Suggested weight: light to medium.

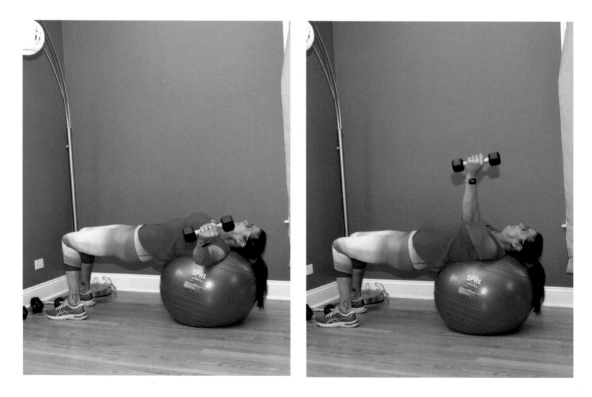

BALL PUSHUP

This exercise requires a lot of balance, so if you have someone nearby who can help, that's an option to consider. Also, you can easily do this on the floor without the ball if you don't feel balanced. Otherwise, kneel on your mat with the ball in front of you and press your hips into the ball. Slowly walk the hands out, balancing on the ball. You can also leave the legs down touching the floor instead of lifting them. The further out you go, the more difficult the move is, so you might want to keep it under your hips for your first go-around. With the hands just wider than shoulder level, lower into a pushup, but avoid bending at the hips. Press back up and repeat for all reps. As a modification, simply practice rolling forward on the ball and back for your first go-around.

   1 x 12 reps

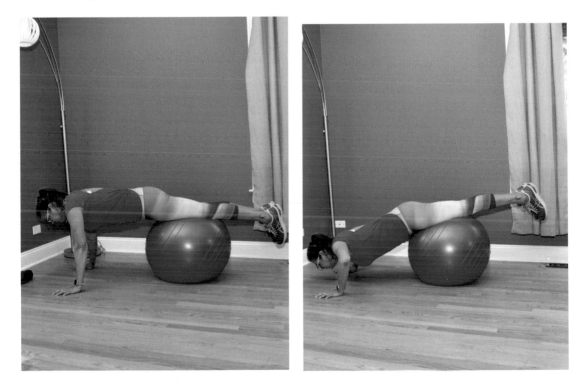

BALL TRICEPS EXTENSIONS

You can do this exercise seated on a ball or chair or as shown. You can hold the weights or place them on a chair next to you if you need more balance. Sit on the ball and slowly walk forward until your back and neck are supported on the ball. Take the weights straight up overhead with the palms facing in. Bend the elbows, lowering the weight to about ear level. Press the weights back up and repeat for all reps. As a modification, stay seated instead of rolling forward, or have your weights on a surface next to you when you get into place. Suggested weight: light to medium.

1 x 12 reps

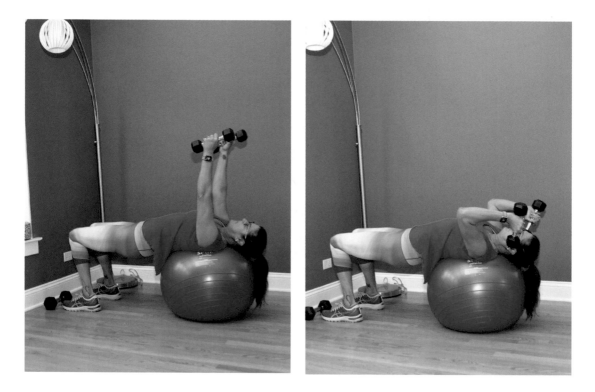

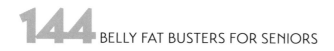

BALL CRUNCHES

Sit on the ball and slowly walk the feet forward until the ball is under your mid-back. Put your hands behind your head and gently support it as you squeeze the abs and lift the shoulders off the ball. To make it easier, you can walk forward and try it at an incline. Lower and repeat for all reps. As modifications, do these without the ball or use a wall to help you walk forward on the ball.

   1 x 12 reps

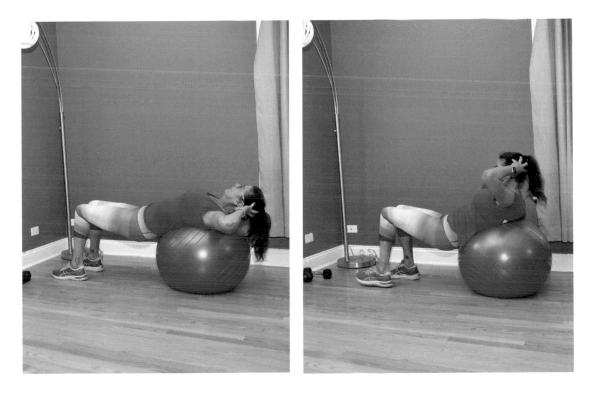

BENT-KNEE BACK EXTENSIONS

You can do these with the ball or on the floor lying flat. If you're using a ball, put it in front of you and lean into it, knees bent and hands behind the head or on the ball for light support. Lift the chest off the ball as you brace your abs. You only need to go up a few inches. Lower back down and repeat for all reps. Again, as a modification, do these on the floor instead of using the ball.

   1 x 12 reps

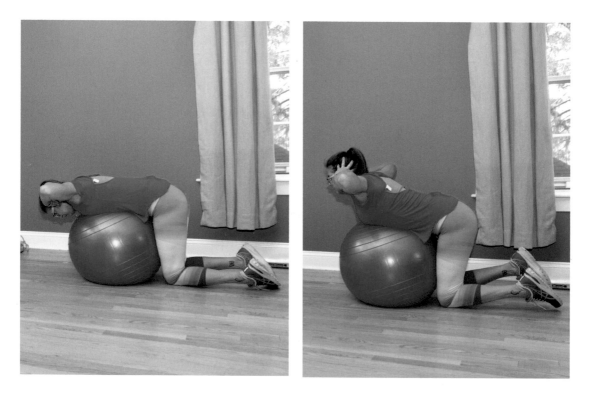

Chapter 13

Weeks 11 & 12—Your Most Challenging Workouts

We're at the finish line, although you know you have to keep going if you want to stay strong, independent, and fit.

The workouts are going to look a little different for the next couple of weeks because I'm adding new equipment: a step. Remember, this is optional. All the exercises can be done on the floor if you don't have a step or don't feel safe using one.

I like adding a step because it ramps up the intensity of your workouts and builds strength, especially in the lower body.

In the workout, I'm using a step with one riser under each side. If you do have a step, you can start with just the platform (usually around four inches) to get used to it. But, again, all of these moves can be done without a step. If you do use one, I recommend keeping it next to a wall or sturdy support for balance as you practice using it, if you haven't used one before.

As with the previous Total Body Circuit Workout, I'm adding a third strength circuit workout to the schedule. It's up to you if you want to add that.

Keep in mind that you don't have to keep to the same schedule every week. Some weeks, you may need to do less and some weeks you'll feel strong enough to do more. That's normal. Our bodies, energy levels, sleep patterns, and more change from day to day, so it's important to give your body what it needs, whether that's more exercise, more sleep, or more stress management.

More importantly, now is a great time to take a breath and think about how far you've come. Whatever you've accomplished, you deserve a pat on the back and a reward. We'll talk about that more in the next chapter.

For now, let's get moving.

SUGGESTED WORKOUT SCHEDULE:

Day 1: Total Body Strength Circuit 6/Cool down
Day 2: Rest and active movement
Day 3: Cardio HIIT or LISS
Day 4: Total Body Strength Circuit 6/Cool down
Day 5: Rest and flexibility
Day 6: Cardio HIIT or LISS and core
Day 7: Total Body Strength Circuit 6/Cool down

The Workout: Total Body Strength Circuit 6
Equipment: Light to heavy dumbbells, a step (optional), a chair, a mat
How it Works: Do each exercise one after the other, completing 1-3 circuits. If you do more than one circuit, rest for about 30 seconds to a minute in between circuits.

SIDE SQUAT OFF STEP
If you're using a step, start on top and towards the right end of the step and hold weights in both hands. Carefully step out onto the floor into a squat to the left of the step, keeping the right foot on the step. Press into the heel to stand up and repeat for all reps before switching sides. As a modification, do the move without a weight or hold the weight in one hand and then hold on to a support for more balance. Suggested weight: light to medium.

 1 x 12 reps

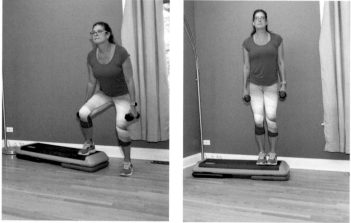

ELEVATED PUSHUP

If you're using a step, place the platform and any risers you're using on the mat. On your knees or toes (harder), place the hands on the step and lower the hips so that your head is in line with your knees. Bend the elbows and lower into a pushup. Press back up to start and repeat for all reps. You may want to use a mat or towel to protect your hands. As a modification, do these on the floor or do a wall pushup.

   1 x 12 reps

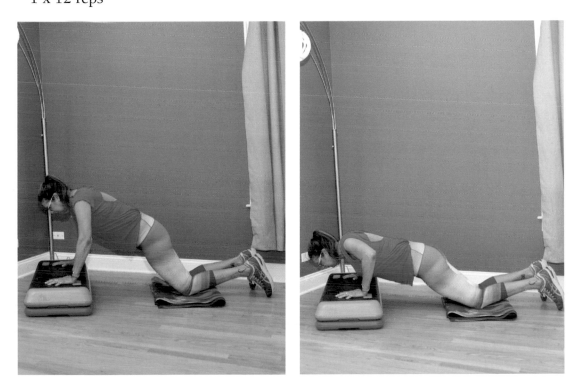

ONE-LEGGED BURPEE

This one is pretty advanced, involving going down to the floor and up again. This is a great move to practice just for your own safety, but can be very challenging. Skip it if you feel like this is a no for you. Stand in front of your step if you're using one—you can also do this on the floor. Squat and place both hands on the step. Take the left leg straight back, then step it back in and stand up. Repeat, alternating sides. For more intensity you can jump at the end, or even jump both feet back at the same time.

   1 x 12 reps

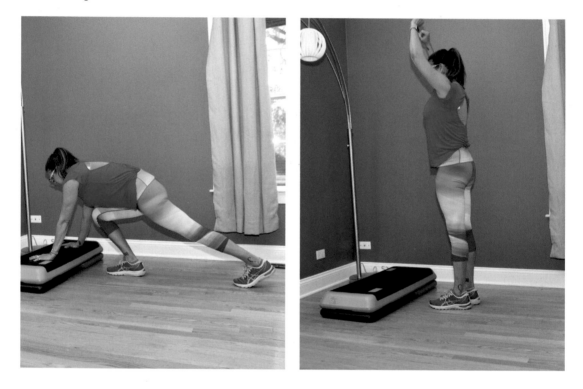

REAR LUNGE OFF THE STEP

You might want to keep a chair or wall handy for balance if you need to. You can also do this move on the floor. If you're using a step, stand on top of the step holding weights. Step off the back of the step with the left leg into a lunge, keeping the front knee at a 90-degree angle. Push into the heel to step back to start and repeat for all reps before switching sides. As modifications, hold on to a wall, don't use weights, or do this on the floor. Suggested weight: light to medium.

1 x 12 reps

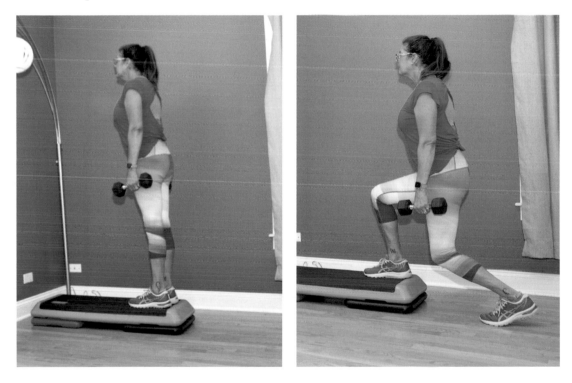

OVERHEAD PRESS

For this exercise, you won't need the step. Hold weights in both hands and stand with feet together, knees slightly bent. Start with the elbows bent and the weight next to the ears. Keeping the abs braced, press the weights overhead, targeting the shoulders. Lower and repeat for all reps. Suggested weight: medium to heavy.

1x12 reps

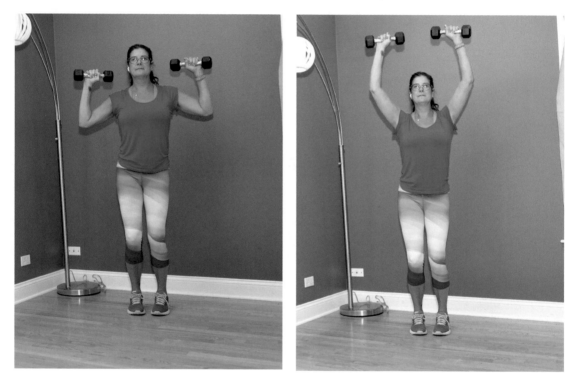

SIT AND STANDS

This move can be done with a chair or, if you want more intensity you can actually use your step. If you're using a chair, put it behind you and sit down to make sure it's in the right position. For the exercise, sit on the chair and take the legs straight out. Bring the legs in, stand up and (optional) jump. The same movements apply if you're using the step, but obviously you're going much further down which will increase the intensity.

1 x 12 reps

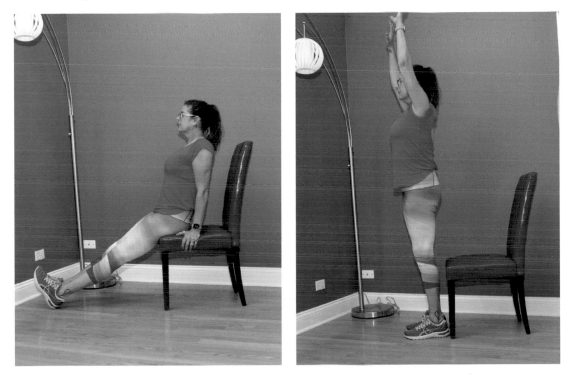

STEP-UPS

Stand in front of the step if you're using one, holding weights in both hands. Step the left foot on the step and press through the heel to step all the way up, bringing the right foot next to the left. Step back down and repeat all reps before switching sides. As a modification, hold a weight in one hand and use the other to hold on to a wall or support for balance. You can also do this move on the floor; you may just want to turn it into a lunge as in previous exercises. Suggested weight: medium to heavy.

1 x 12 reps

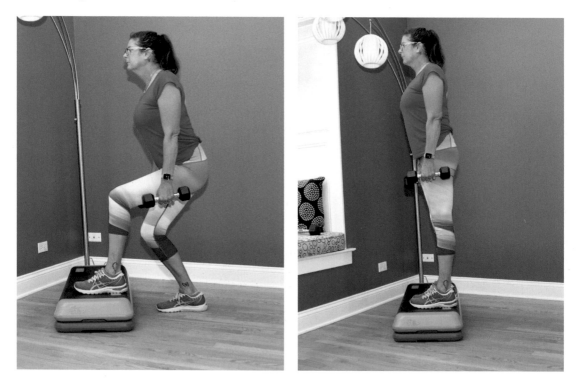

BICEPS CURLS 21s

For these biceps curls, you're going to do something called 21s. Hold weights in both hands and curl the weights halfway up. Lower down and repeat for 7 reps. After 7 reps, start halfway up and curl the weights all the way up. Continue for 7 reps, going up and halfway down. For your last set of 7 reps, you'll go all the way up and all the way down. Changing the tempo makes the exercise different and can increase intensity. Suggested weight: medium to heavy.

1 x 21 reps

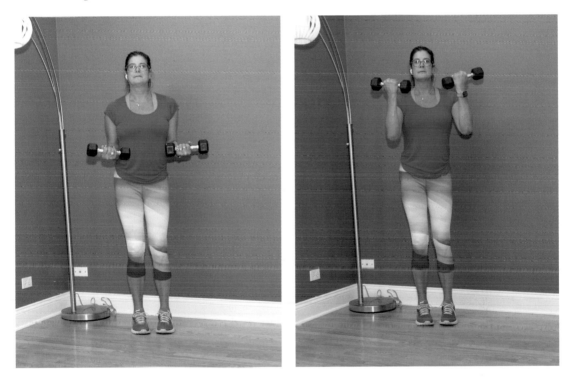

SQUAT AND REACH CARDIO

We're inserting a little cardio here with the squat and reach, which you've done before. Squat as low as you can, crossing the arms in front of the knees. Stand and take the arms up and out. You can also add a jump if you want more intensity. Repeat for 30 seconds or about 16 reps.

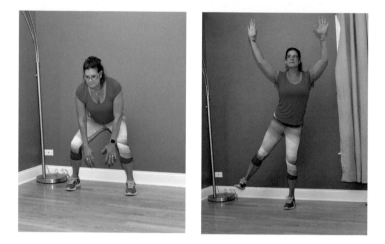

SIDE LUNGE CURL

Hold a weight in the right hand and step out into a side lunge with the right leg. The right leg should be straight. Take the weight as low to the floor as you can. Press into the heel to stand up, bringing the feet together and curling the weight up towards the shoulder. Repeat for all reps before switching sides. Suggested weight: medium to heavy.

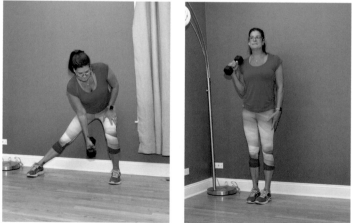

PULLOVER WITH CHEST FLY

You can do this move on the step or on the floor. Lie down and hold weights in both hands straight up over the chest. Press the weights together and, with the elbows bent and the abs engaged, slowly drop the arms behind you to about step level. Squeeze your back to lift the weights back up and then open the hands, taking both arms out to the sides in a chest fly. If the pullover doesn't feel good, just stick with the flies. As a modification, just do the flies, or do the moves separately. The pullovers really require you to brace your core, so make sure your back doesn't hurt during this exercise. Suggested weight: light to medium.

1 x 12 reps (1 rep includes a pullover and a fly)

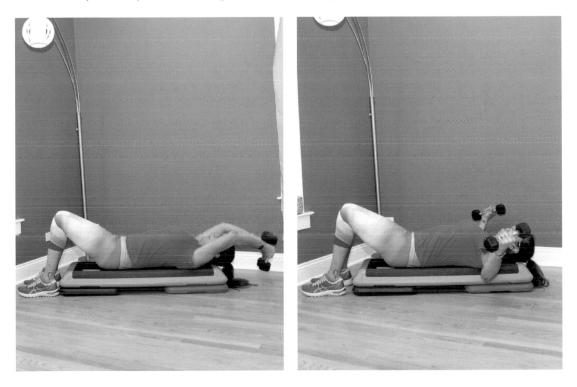

KNEE SMASH

With the weight on the right leg and arms straight up at a diagonal, pull the left knee up towards the chest while bringing the arms down and squeezing the abs. Repeat as fast as you can for 30 seconds and switch sides. You can add a jump if you want a higher intensity. As a modification, you can hold onto a wall and just use one arm in your knee smash.

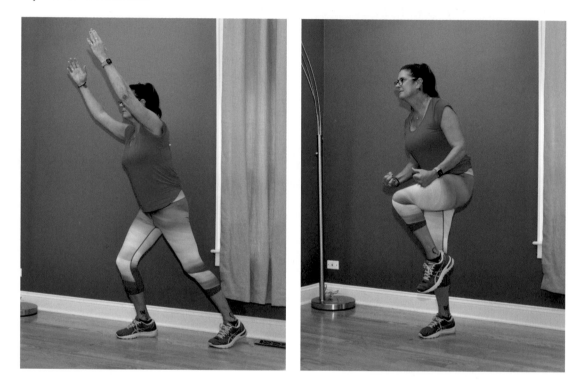

STEP UP LEG LIFT

If you're using a step, hold weights in both hands and make your way to the right side of the step. Starting on top, step to the floor with the left foot, lowering into a squat. As you press back up, lift the left leg up in a leg lift. As a modification, just hold one weight and use the other hand to hold on to a wall or support for balance. You can also take the leg lift out. Lower and repeat for all reps before switching sides. Suggested weight: light to medium.

   1 x 12 reps

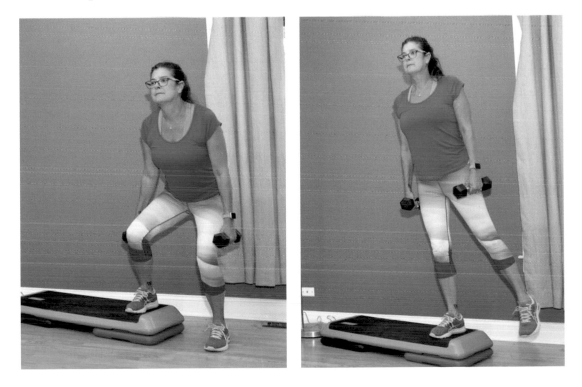

KICKBACKS

Hold weights in both hands and tip from the hips with the back flat and abs into about a 45-degree angle. Begin the move with the elbows bent, weights in, and then extend the arms back, squeezing the triceps. Lower and repeat for all reps. As a modification, hold one weight and, as you tip from the hips, use the other hand on your thigh for more back support. Do the reps on one side and then switch. Suggested weight: light to medium.

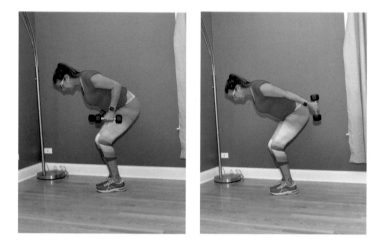

STEP OUTS WITH OVERHEAD REACH

Keep the weight on the right leg and step out with the left foot while raising the left arm up at a diagonal. Go as fast as you can for 30 seconds and repeat on the other side.

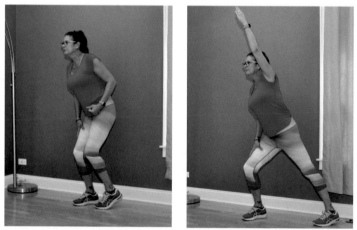

Chapter 14

What Happens Now?

The end of this book does not mean it's the end of your workouts. It's just like everything else you do in life. You have to keep doing it or you lose all the gains you've made . . . or losses, if you've lost some weight.

At this point, I hope it's become more of a habit for you and something that, just maybe, you actually look forward to.

But, there are some things to keep in mind as you move forward. These workouts are a great start, but you always want to keep challenging yourself with new activities and different ways to lift weights.

I have some tips to keep you going and help you change things up so that you keep building more strength and fitness.

HOW TO CHANGE YOUR WORKOUTS

There are a variety of elements of your workouts that you can manipulate to make things more interesting and to challenge your muscles. Just a few include:

✓ **Your Reps**: throughout this book, I've kept the reps at about 12 for most exercises, but you're not limited by that. In fact, the general guidelines suggest anywhere from 4 to 16 reps, so you have a range to work within. Here's one way to approach this:
  » Start with 12 reps of an exercise
  » When 12 feels easy, add on more reps until you get to 16 reps
  » If you can do more than 16 reps, increase the weight and drop the reps down—You can choose 8, 10, or 12. The idea is that, the fewer reps you do, the heavier your weights will be.

- ✓ **Your Weights**: as you can see above, changing your weights is something that will happen naturally if you're paying attention to how you feel and getting stronger. You can also change the type of resistance you're using including:
  - » Resistance bands
  - » Barbells
  - » Kettlebells
  - » Gym machines
  - » Medicine balls or even sandbags
- ✓ **Your Exercises**: if you look through the program, you'll see how the exercises change every couple of weeks. It's a great idea to mix things up, especially once you get so many weeks under your belt. It may take a little research, but here are a few things you can do to change what you're doing:
  - » **Do one limb at a time**: For example, instead of squats, do a one-legged squat and hold on to the wall for balance if needed. Stand on one foot to do things like biceps curls or triceps extensions.
  - » **Use an exercise ball**: You'll see from many of the workouts that an exercise ball can be used for a variety of moves. Feel free to experiment with squats, lunges (putting the back foot on the ball), crunches with a medicine ball, or rotating from side to side. You can also get into an incline position on the ball and do things like biceps curls or front raises for the shoulders. This builds coordination and core strength. Just make sure you feel safe before using a weight.
  - » **Change your position**: One thing about strength training is that you want to move against gravity, but choosing different types of equipment means you can get in different positions. For example, you can do a chest press on the floor with dumbbells, but if you want to work your chest while standing up, you can use resistance bands or a cable machine.
  - » **Change the type of resistance**: I've talked about everything from dumbbells and resistance bands, to kettlebells and machines. The trick here is to first know which body part you're working. Then

you can do some research (or use the ideas in this book) to find new ways to work, say, your chest, or your back.

» **Do something totally different**: It's easy to get into a rut with exercise, so think of ways to make things more interesting. Maybe train for a 5K, take a group fitness class, or walk with a friend. Doing the same thing over and over gets boring and sometimes that might affect your motivation and momentum.

» **Always keep moving:** Remember that everything counts, whether you walk for five minutes or lift weights for an hour. Don't feel like you have to workout for a certain amount of time if you don't have the time or energy. Just do something!

TAKING AN EXERCISE BREAK

Something many exercisers like to do is to take about a week off every three or so months. This is a great way to let your body rest and replenish your energy stores, although some people worry about losing what they've gained.

Here are some signs you may need an exercise break:

✓ **You feel tired or burned out**—This program includes a lot of exercises, and there are times when your body just needs a break. If you're dreading your workout, give yourself some time off or do something simple like walking or stretching.

✓ **You have a nagging pain**—We've all had that experience when something hurts just enough to be annoying. Don't ignore that. It could be a sign that you're overdoing it or maybe doing something too repetitive. This is a time to stop, perhaps try other activities, or even see your doctor. Being proactive means you don't have to take time out for an injury you could avoid.

✓ **You're losing sleep**—There are times when you have to make choices and sometimes it's a choice between exercise and sleep. As a young person, I didn't even consider that an option. As I get older? Sleep becomes extremely precious. If you're not sleeping great, don't worry if you decide to skip workouts because you just need more sleep.

✓ **You have a chronic injury**—I know that I've made the mistake of working through the pain, which is code for doing something dumb. Working through any kind of pain—remember this is sharp pain in the joints or muscles, not just muscle soreness—puts you at risk for a chronic injury that can haunt you. It's no fun going to the doctor, but it's the best thing you can do for your health when you're experiencing this kind of pain.

The point is, exercise helps you get to know yourself and your body. The trick is to listen to what's happening and make good decisions so you can keep moving and avoid injury. It's a tall order, I know, but you do get more intuitive as you move your body on a consistent basis.

WHAT HAPPENS WHEN YOU TAKE A BREAK

With all of that said about taking a break, many of my clients wonder what happens to your fitness if you stop exercising.

First, I'll tell you that taking a week off won't really affect your endurance or strength. You may feel a little stiff as you come back to exercise, but you're nor really losing any of your fitness.

Beyond that, you can lose some fitness, but the most important thing to remember is that you can always get it back. Muscle memory is a real thing. Your body will always remember these exercises; it may just take time to build back your muscle and endurance.

So, what really happens if you stop exercising for a longer period of time? Just some things to think about:

✓ Your cardio endurance can decline about 5 to 10 percent in three weeks.
✓ It takes about two months of inactivity to lose all the gains you've made after you've done a full 12-week program.
✓ You do have muscle memory, which means your body will remember the movements even if you've taking a break.

The good news is, it's never too late to start exercising, whether you've taken a break or you're just getting started. We're all capable of improving ourselves as long as we're patient, we listen to our bodies, and we do what feels right.

The most important thing you can do for yourself is to never give up!

Resources

"5 Benefits of Compound Exercises." Accessed September 14, 2021. https://www.acefitness.org/education-and-resources/professional/expert-articles/5811/5-benefits-of-compound-exercises/.

Bulun, S. E., K. Zeitoun, H. Sasano, and E. R. Simpson. "Aromatase in Aging Women." *Seminars in Reproductive Endocrinology* 17, no. 4 (1999): 349–58. https://doi.org/10.1055/s-2007-1016244.

Cheung, Karoline, Patria Hume, and Linda Maxwell. "Delayed Onset Muscle Soreness: Treatment Strategies and Performance Factors." *Sports Medicine* 33, no. 2 (2003): 145–64. https://doi.org/10.2165/00007256-200333020-00005.

Cleary, Michelle A, Michael R Sitler, and Zebulon V Kendrick. "Dehydration and Symptoms of Delayed-Onset Muscle Soreness in Normothermic Men." *Journal of Athletic Training* 41, no. 1 (2006): 36–45.

Davis, S. R., C. Castelo-Branco, P. Chedraui, M. A. Lumsden, R. E. Nappi, D. Shah, and P Villaseca. "Understanding Weight Gain at Menopause." *Climacteric* 15, no. 5 (October 2012): 419–29. https://doi.org/10.3109/13697137.2012.707385.

Dillaway, Heather E. "When Does Menopause Occur, and How Long Does It Last? Wrestling with Age- and Time-Based Conceptualizations of Reproductive Aging." *NWSA Journal* 18, no. 1 (2006): 31–60.

Garber, Carol Ewing, Bryan Blissmer, Michael R. Deschenes, Barry A. Franklin, Michael J. Lamonte, I.-Min Lee, David C. Nieman, David P. Swain. "American College of Sports Medicine Position Stand. Quantity and Quality of Exercise for Developing and Maintaining Cardiorespiratory, Musculoskeletal, and Neuromotor Fitness in Apparently Healthy Adults: Guidance for Prescribing Exercise." *Medicine & Science in Sports & Exercise* 43, no. 7 (July 2011): 1334–59. https://doi.org/10.1249/MSS.0b013e318213fefb.

Greer, Beau Kjerulf, Prawee Sirithienthad, Robert J. Moffatt, Richard T. Marcello, and Lynn B. Panton. "EPOC Comparison Between Isocaloric Bouts of Steady-State Aerobic, Intermittent Aerobic, and Resistance Training." *Research Quarterly for Exercise and Sport* 86, no. 2 (April 3, 2015): 190–95. https://doi.org/10.1080/02701367.2014.999190.

Henderson, Victor W. "Cognitive Changes After Menopause: Influence of Estrogen." *Clinical Obstetrics and Gynecology* 51, no. 3 (September 2008): 618–26. https://doi.org/10.1097/GRF.0b013e318180ba10.

"How Do I Know I'm in Menopause? " Accessed September 15, 2021. https://www.menopause.org/for-women/menopauseflashes/menopause-symptoms-and-treatments/how-do-i-know-when-i'm-in-menopause-.

"How Does Menopause Affect My Sleep?" Accessed September 15, 2021. https://www.hopkinsmedicine.org/health/wellness-and-prevention/how-does-menopause-affect-my-sleep.

"Intestinal Obstruction—Symptoms and Causes." Accessed October 16, 2021. https://www.mayoclinic.org/diseases-conditions/intestinal-obstruction/symptoms-causes/syc-20351460.

Irving, Brian A., Christopher K. Davis, David W. Brock, Judy Y. Weltman, Damon Swift, Eugene J. Barrett, Glenn A. Gaesser, and Arthur Weltman. "Effect of Exercise Training Intensity on Abdominal Visceral Fat and Body Composition." *Medicine & Science in Sports & Exercise* 40, no. 11 (November 2008): 1863–72. https://doi.org/10.1249/MSS.0b013e3181801d40.

Jehan, Shazia, Alina Masters-Isarilov, Idoko Salifu, Ferdinand Zizi, Girardin Jean-Louis, Seithikurippu R Pandi-Perumal, Ravi Gupta, Amnon Brzezinski, and Samy I McFarlane. "Sleep Disorders in Postmenopausal Women." *Journal of Sleep Disorders & Therapy* 4, no. 5 (August 2015): 212.

Joffe, Hadine, Katherine A. Guthrie, Andrea Z. LaCroix, Susan D. Reed, Kristine E. Ensrud, JoAnn E. Manson, Katherine M. Newton, et al. "Low-Dose Estradiol and the Serotonin-Norepinephrine Reuptake Inhibitor Venlafaxine for Vasomotor Symptoms: A Randomized Clinical Trial." *JAMA Internal Medicine* 174, no. 7 (July 1, 2014): 1058–66. https://doi.org/10.1001/jamainternmed.2014.1891.

Keating, Shelley E., Elizabeth A. Machan, Helen T. O'Connor, James A. Gerofi, Amanda Sainsbury, Ian D. Caterson, and Nathan A. Johnson. "Continuous Exercise but Not High Intensity Interval Training Improves Fat Distribution in Overweight Adults." *Journal of Obesity* 2014 (January 16, 2014): e834865. https://doi.org/10.1155/2014/834865.

Kovacevic, Ana, Yorgi Mavros, Jennifer J. Heisz, and Maria A. Fiatarone Singh. "The Effect of Resistance Exercise on Sleep: A Systematic Review of Randomized Controlled Trials." *Sleep Medicine Reviews* 39 (June 2018): 52–68. https://doi.org/10.1016/j.smrv.2017.07.002.

Laforgia, J., R. T. Withers, and C. J. Gore. "Effects of Exercise Intensity and Duration on the Excess Post-Exercise Oxygen Consumption." *Journal of Sports Sciences* 24, no. 12 (December 1, 2006): 1247–64. https://doi.org/10.1080/02640410600552064.

Lee, Jinju, Youngsin Han, Hyun Hee Cho, and Mee-Ran Kim. "Sleep Disorders and Menopause." *Journal of Menopausal Medicine* 25, no. 2 (August 2019): 83–87. https://doi.org/10.6118/jmm.19192.

Lucas, Rebekah A. I. "Is Exercise an Effective Therapy for Menopause and Hot Flashes?" *Menopause* 23, no. 7 (July 2016): 701–3. https://doi.org/10.1097/GME.0000000000000707.

Maki, Pauline M., and Victor W. Henderson. "Cognition and the Menopause Transition." *Menopause* 23, no. 7 (July 2016): 803–5. https://doi.org/10.1097/GME.0000000000000681.

Mattes, R. D. and W. W. Campbell. "Effects of Food Form and Timing of Ingestion on Appetite and Energy Intake in Lean and Obese Young Adults." *Journal of the American Dietetic Association* 109, no. 3 (March 2009): 430–37. https://doi.org/10.1016/j.jada.2008.11.031.

"Menopause and Libido: Does Menopause Affect Sex Drive?," May 9, 2017. https://www.healthline.com/health/menopause/menopause-libido.

Milanović, Zoran, Saša Pantelić, Nebojša Trajković, Goran Sporiš, Radmila Kostić, and Nic James. "Age-Related Decrease in Physical Activity and Functional Fitness among Elderly Men and Women." *Clinical Interventions in Aging* 8 (2013): 549–56. https://doi.org/10.2147/CIA.S44112.

Mishra, Nalini, V. N. Mishra, and Devanshi. "Exercise beyond Menopause. Dos and Don'ts." *Journal of Mid-Life Health* 2, no. 2 (2011): 51–56. https://doi.org/10.4103/0976-7800.92524.

Mulhall, Stephanie, Ross Andel, and Kaarin J. Anstey. "Variation in Symptoms of Depression and Anxiety in Midlife Women by Menopausal Status." *Maturitas* 108 (February 2018): 7–12. https://doi.org/10.1016/j.maturitas.2017.11.005.

Newsom, Rob. "How Blue Light Affects Sleep," Sleep Foundation, November 4, 2020. https://www.sleepfoundation.org/bedroom-environment/blue-light.

Paoli, Antonio, Andrea Casolo, Matteo Saoncella, Carlo Bertaggia, Marco Fantin, Antonino Bianco, Giuseppe Marcolin, and Tatiana Moro. "Effect of an Endurance and Strength Mixed Circuit Training on Regional Fat Thickness: The Quest for the 'Spot Reduction.'" *International Journal of Environmental Research and Public Health* 18, no. 7 (January 2021): 3845. https://doi.org/10.3390/ijerph18073845.

 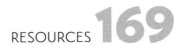

Peterson, Mark D., Ananda Sen, and Paul M. Gordon. "Influence of Resistance Exercise on Lean Body Mass in Aging Adults: A Meta-Analysis." *Medicine & Science in Sports & Exercise* 43, no. 2 (February 2011): 249–58. https://doi.org/10.1249/MSS.0b013e3181eb6265.

Pinkerton, JoAnn V., Hadine Joffe, Kazem Kazempour, Hana Mekonnen, Sailaja Bhaskar, and Joel Lippman. "Low-Dose Paroxetine (7.5 Mg) Improves Sleep in Women with Vasomotor Symptoms Associated with Menopause." *Menopause* 22, no. 1 (January 2015): 50–58. https://doi.org/10.1097/GME.0000000000000311.

Plangger, Kirk, Colin Campbell, Karen Robson, and Matteo Montecchi. "Little Rewards, Big Changes: Using Exercise Analytics to Motivate Sustainable Changes in Physical Activity." *Information & Management*, November 2, 2019, 103216. https://doi.org/10.1016/j.im.2019.103216.

Polidori, David, Arjun Sanghvi, Randy J. Seeley, and Kevin D. Hall. "How Strongly Does Appetite Counter Weight Loss? Quantification of the Feedback Control of Human Energy Intake." *Obesity* 24, no. 11 (2016): 2289–95. https://doi.org/10.1002/oby.21653.

Rodgers, Jennifer L., Jarrod Jones, Samuel I. Bolleddu, Sahit Vanthenapalli, Lydia E. Rodgers, Kinjal Shah, Krishna Karia, and Siva K. Panguluri. "Cardiovascular Risks Associated with Gender and Aging." *Journal of Cardiovascular Development and Disease* 6, no. 2 (April 27, 2019): 19. https://doi.org/10.3390/jcdd6020019.

Romano, Antonino D., Gaetano Serviddio, Angela de Matthaeis, Francesco Bellanti, and Gianluigi Vendemiale. "Oxidative Stress and Aging." *Journal of Nephrology* 23 Suppl 15 (September 1, 2010): S29-36.

Romero-Arenas, Salvador, Miryam Martínez-Pascual, and Pedro E. Alcaraz. "Impact of Resistance Circuit Training on Neuromuscular, Cardiorespiratory and Body Composition Adaptations in the Elderly." *Aging and Disease* 4, no. 5 (October 1, 2013): 256–63. https://doi.org/10.14336/AD.2013.0400256.

Siu, Parco M., Angus P. Yu, Edwin C. Chin, Doris S. Yu, Stanley S. Hui, Jean Woo, Daniel Y. Fong, Gao X. Wei, and Michael R. Irwin. "Effects of Tai Chi or Conventional Exercise on Central Obesity in Middle-Aged and Older Adults." *Annals of Internal Medicine* 174, no. 8 (August 17, 2021): 1050–57. https://doi.org/10.7326/M20-7014.

"Symptoms of Menopause at Every Age: 40 to 65." Accessed September 15, 2021. https://www.healthline.com/health/menopause/symptoms-of-menopause.

"The Physical Activity Guidelines for Americans" Accessed September 20, 2021. https://jamanetwork.com/journals/jama/article-abstract/2712935.

US News & World Report. "Estrogen Loss Is a Main Driver of Fat Gain, Studies Show." Accessed September 15, 2021. https://health.usnews.com/wellness/articles/2018-04-06/what-causes-menopausal-belly-fat.

Van Aggel-Leijssen, Dorien P. van, Wim H. Saris, Anton J. Wagenmakers, Gabby B. Hul, and Marleen A. van Baak. "The Effect of Low-Intensity Exercise Training on Fat Metabolism of Obese Women." *Obesity* 9, no. 2 (2001): 86–96. https://doi.org/10.1038/oby.2001.11.

Walston, Jeremy D. "Sarcopenia in Older Adults." *Current Opinion in Rheumatology* 24, no. 6 (November 2012): 623–27. https://doi.org/10.1097/BOR.0b013e328358d59b.

Wojtek J. Chodzko-Zajko, David N. Proctor, Maria A. Fiatarone Singh, Christopher T. Minson, Claudio R. Nigg, George J. Salem, and James S. Skinner. "American College of Sports Medicine Position Stand. Exercise and Physical Activity for Older Adults." *Medicine & Science in Sports & Exercise* 41, no. 7 (July 2009): 1510–30. https://doi.org/10.1249/MSS.0b013e3181a0c95c.

Wolkove, Norman, Osama Elkholy, Marc Baltzan, and Mark Palayew. "Sleep and Aging: 1. Sleep Disorders Commonly Found in Older People." *CMAJ* 176, no. 9 (April 24, 2007): 1299–1304. https://doi.org/10.1503/cmaj.060792.

Zeng, Tian, Jing Zhao, Yu Kang, Xiaojiao Wang, and Hongjun Xie. "Association between Polymorphism near the MC4R Gene and Cancer Risk: A Meta-Analysis." *Medicine* 99, no. 36 (September 4, 2020): e22003. https://doi.org/10.1097/MD.0000000000022003.